# Reproductive Tract Infections

## Reproductive Health Epidemiology Series
## Module 3

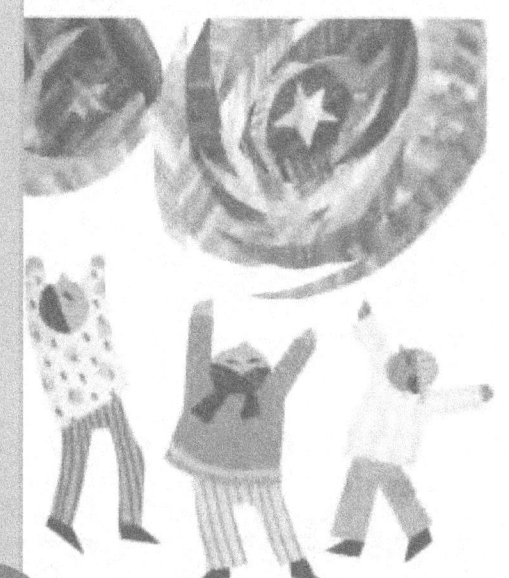

**2003**

DEPARTMENT OF HEALTH AND HUMAN SERVICES

# REPRODUCTIVE TRACT INFECTIONS

REPRODUCTIVE HEALTH
EPIDEMIOLOGY SERIES:
MODULE 3

June 2003

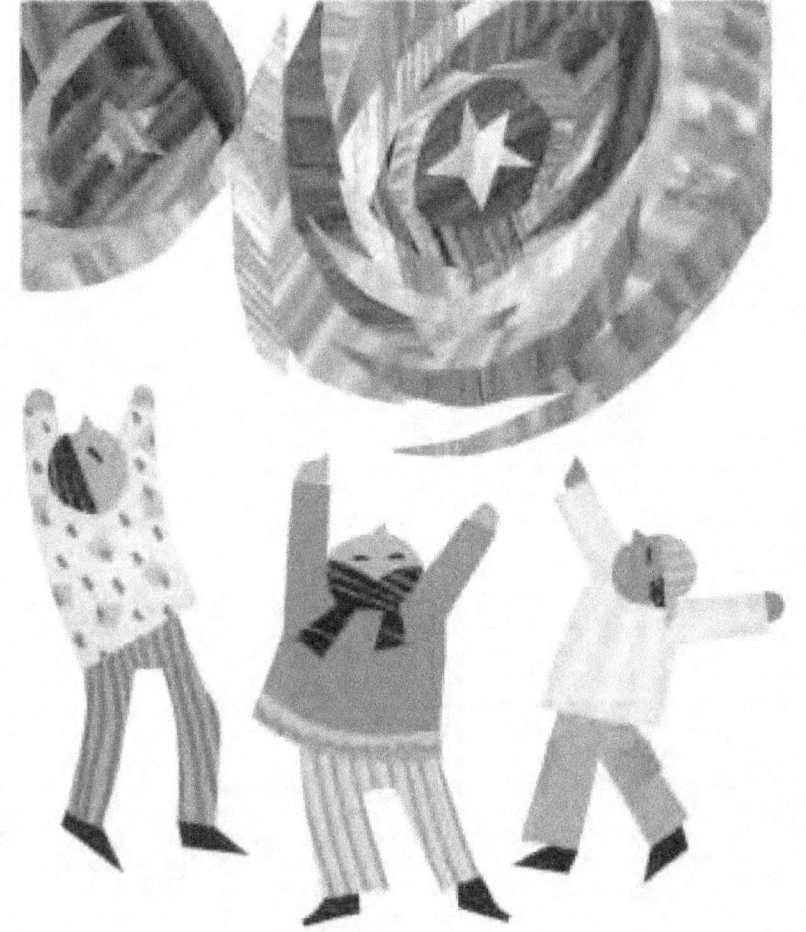

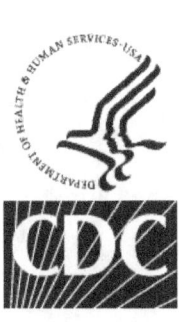

The United States Agency for International Development (USAID) provided funding for this project through a Participating Agency Service Agreement with CDC (936-3038.01).

# REPRODUCTIVE TRACT INFECTIONS

Divya A. Patel, MPH
Nancy M. Burnett, BS
Kathryn M. Curtis, PhD

**Technical Editors**
Susan Hillis, PhD
Polly Marchbanks, PhD

U.S. Department of Health and Human Services
Centers for Disease Control and Prevention
National Center for Chronic Disease Prevention and Health Promotion
Division of Reproductive Health
Atlanta, Georgia, U.S.A.
2003

# CONTENTS

# REPRODUCTIVE TRACT INFECTIONS

## LEARNING OBJECTIVES

This module is designed for reproductive health professionals interested in conducting surveillance and epidemiologic studies related to reproductive tract infections (RTIs) and who need a working knowledge of epidemiologic and analytic issues specific to RTIs.

After studying the material in this module, the student should be able to:

- Identify the major viral and bacterial RTIs and their sequelae.

- Describe the interaction between reproductive tract infections and family planning, child survival, safe motherhood, and HIV prevention.

- Understand the general model for the spread of infection and its implications in the control and prevention of RTIs.

- Translate the general model for the spread of infection into practical biologic and behavioral determinants of the spread of infection.

- Describe how data from surveillance systems and epidemiologic studies can be linked to public health action to reduce the burden of RTIs.

- Understand the major epidemiologic and analytic issues specific to RTIs.

- Describe the uses of research and collected data, including the dissemination of findings.

## Case Study: Reproductive Tract Infections—Ethiopia

*The prevalence of reproductive tract infections (RTIs) in Ethiopia is among the highest in Africa. Despite a decrease in the prevalence of syphilis since the 1960s due to increased use of antibiotics, the number of cases of gonorrhea, chancroid, and lymphogranuloma venereum reported to the Ministry of Health increased three to five times between 1983 and 1990.*

*Recognizing the cultural, social, and economic barriers for women attending sexually transmitted disease (STD) clinics in the face of this growing public health problem, researchers became interested in exploring possibilities for interventions in health services routinely attended by Ethiopian women. A study was conducted among 542 women attending family planning clinics (FPCs) and 1,569 women attending gynecological outpatient departments (GOPDs) to examine the socioeconomic and cultural context of family planning and to determine the prevalence of certain RTIs, pelvic inflammatory disease (PID), and cervical cancer among both groups of women.*

*A full abdominal and gynecological examination, along with a questionnaire soliciting detailed demographic and lifestyle information, was administered to each woman in the study. Clinical examinations revealed that, although women attending FPCs had fewer symptoms than those attending GOPDs, they had more clinical evidence of past and present PID and more active infections requiring immediate treatment. Serological testing revealed that these women also had more evidence of exposure to STDs with higher titers indicative of active or present infection. Of particular concern, only 4% of women attending FPCs had no serological evidence of RTIs, and 64% had serological evidence of three or more different infections. Use of FPC services was found to be associated with higher levels of income and education; therefore, broadening educational opportunities for girls and women should increase acceptance of FPC services and bring about more opportunities for detection, treatment, and prevention of RTIs.*

*A significant implication of this study is that targeting women who attend FPCs for epidemiologic studies and control and prevention programs is an effective way to reach women who, for various reasons, may not attend STD clinics. The FPC visit provides an opportunity for screening women who are particularly at risk for infection and for educating women about modes of STD transmission and prevention of future infection. When treatment for RTIs can be offered in the FPC, women are not required to make separate visits to other primary health centers for care. On the basis of studies such as this one, adequate screening, treatment, and education of women attending FPCs and their partners should be considered as ways of easing the burden of RTIs in the community.*

*Adapted from: Duncan ME, Tibaux G, Kloos H, et al. STDs in women attending family planning clinics: a case study in Addis Ababa. Soc Sci Med 1997;44(4):441–54.*

# OVERVIEW OF REPRODUCTIVE TRACT INFECTIONS

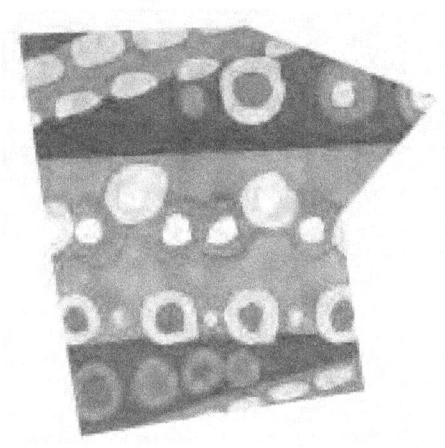

Reproductive tract infections (RTIs) include three types of infection: 1) sexually transmitted diseases (STDs), such as chlamydia, gonorrhea, chancroid, and human immunodeficiency virus (HIV); 2) endogenous infections, which are caused by overgrowth of organisms normally present in the genital tract of healthy women, such as bacterial vaginosis or vulvovaginal candidiasis; and 3) iatrogenic infections, which are associated with improperly performed medical procedures such as unsafe abortion or poor delivery practices *(1)*. RTIs are preventable, and many are treatable as well.

The burden of untreated RTIs is especially heavy for women because these infections are often asymptomatic or the symptoms are not recognizable. Morbidity and mortality related to RTIs deprive society of important contributions made by women in terms of economic, social, and cultural development. Although RTIs affect women in both developing and industrialized countries, the infections and their sequelae are an especially urgent public health problem in resource-poor areas around the world. Demographic changes in developing countries have led to a dramatic increase in the number of adolescent and young adult women and men in their most sexually active years, which translates into a greater proportion of the population at risk for RTIs. The large number of infants and children in these countries means that this trend will continue for several decades. The risk of RTIs is compounded by rapid urbanization and high male-to-female ratios in some regions *(1)*. The problems associated with RTIs have become even more significant in the past decade with the emergence of HIV and acquired immunodeficiency syndrome (AIDS).

## Prevalence of RTIs

Epidemiologic data show that the incidence and prevalence of various RTIs vary greatly between countries and even between regions within a country, a reflection of the differences in the characteristics of each pathogen (such as duration of infectivity and transmissibility) as well as other biological, behavioral, medical, social, and economic factors *(2)*. Among pregnant women in developing countries, it is estimated that gonorrhea rates are 10–15 times higher, chlamydia rates are 2–3 times higher, and syphilis rates are 10–100 times higher than the rates for these STDs among women in industrialized countries *(1)*. However, because of differences in study design, reporting, specimen collection, and laboratory methods across the world, it is difficult to interpret data on the prevalence of RTIs in developing regions in terms of internal validity or generalizability *(1)*. Still, the data that are available suggest that RTIs are common in almost all of the developing countries in which they have been investigated. Rates of RTIs tend to be highest among high-risk groups such as commercial sex workers and clients of STD clinics, but are also prevalent in asymptomatic populations and low-risk women, such as those attending antenatal clinics *(3)*.

## What Are the Most Commonly Occurring RTIs in Developing Countries?

Some of the more common bacterial infections occurring in developing countries include gonorrhea, chlamydia, syphilis, bacterial vaginosis (BV), lymphogranuloma venereum (LGV), trichomoniasis, and chancroid. Viral infections most common to developing countries include human papillomavirus (HPV), hepatitis B virus (HBV), herpes genitalis (herpes simplex virus [HSV], primarily type HSV-2), and HIV. The pathogens, symptoms, diagnoses, and treatment regimens for the most commonly occurring RTIs in developing countries are listed in Appendix A.

## Sequelae of Untreated RTIs

RTIs and their sequelae have widespread effects on the health and well-being of men, women, young people, and newborns. RTIs can pose a threat to a man's fertility since certain untreated infections, such as *Neisseria gonorrhoeae* or *Chlamydia trachomatis*, can block the *vas deferentia* or cause epididymitis, an inflammation of the tubes through which sperm move from the testes to the *vas deferentia*. Although the dangers to men's reproductive health must be recognized, women are clearly at greater risk of infection and carry the greater burden of the disease. Each year thousands of women die from the sequelae of undiagnosed or untreated RTIs, including cervical cancer, ectopic pregnancy, acute and chronic infections of the uterus and fallopian tubes, and puerperal infections. Other sequelae include infertility, fetal wastage, low birth weight, infant blindness, neonatal pneumonia, and mental retardation. Table 1 outlines the major STD pathogens that produce RTIs, along with pregnancy-associated and chronic conditions caused by these pathogens.

**Table 1. Major STD Pathogens That Produce RTIs and Associated Conditions**

| Agent | Acute Disease | Pregnancy-Associated Conditions | Chronic Conditions |
|---|---|---|---|
| *Neisseria gonorrhoeae* | Urethritis<br>Cervicitis<br>Salpingitis<br>Postpartum endometritis | Prematurity<br>Septic abortion<br>Ophthalmia | Infertility<br>Ectopic pregnancy |
| *Chlamydia trachomatis* | Urethritis<br>Cervicitis<br>Salpingitis | Ophthalmia<br>Pneumonia<br>Postpartum endometritis | Infertility<br>Ectopic pregnancy |
| *Treponema pallidum* | Primary and secondary syphilis | Spontaneous abortion<br>Stillbirth<br>Congenital syphilis | Neurosyphilis<br>Cardiovascular syphilis<br>Gumma |
| *Haemophilus ducreyi* | Genital ulcer | None known | Impotence |
| Human immunodeficiency virus (HIV) | Mononucleosis syndrome | Prematurity<br>Stillbirth<br>Perinatal HIV | AIDS |
| Human papillomavirus (HPV) | Genital warts | Laryngeal papillomatosis | Genital cancer |
| Herpes simplex virus 2 (HSV-2) | Genital ulcer | Neonatal HSV<br>Prematurity | Genital cancer |
| Hepatitis B virus (HBV) | Acute hepatitis | Perinatal HBV | Chronic hepatitis<br>Cirrhosis<br>Hepatoma<br>Vasculitis |

Adapted from: Brunham RC, Embree JE. Sexually transmitted diseases: current and future dimensions of the problem in the third world. In: Germain A, Holmes KK, Piot P, Wasserheit JN, editors. Reproductive tract infections: global impact and priorities for women's reproductive health. New York: Plenum Press; 1992. p. 37.

Policymakers and health care professionals concerned about child survival must address RTIs because of the significant role they play in fetal wastage, low birth weight, and congenital and perinatal infections. The impact of RTIs on pregnancy depends upon the pathogen involved, the chronicity of infection, and the stage of gestation during time of infection *(1)*. In general, RTIs appear to pose a much greater problem in pregnant adolescents than in older pregnant women, who are more likely to be involved in a stable, monogamous relationship at the time of conception *(4)*. The availability of inexpensive, efficacious interventions for several RTIs during pregnancy has led to increased

## Complications and Sequelae of Reproductive Tract Infections and HIV

**Pelvic inflammatory disease (PID)** *A potentially life-threatening condition resulting from complications of* N. gonorrhoea *and* C. trachomatis *infections. PID comprises a spectrum of inflammatory disorders of the upper female genital tract, including any combination of endometritis, salpingitis, tubo-ovarian abscess, and pelvic peritonitis. PID increases the risk of tubal infertility, ectopic pregnancy, and chronic abdominal pain.*

**Tubal infertility** *Associated with PID and results from inflammation and scarring of the fallopian tubes following ascent of gonorrhoea, chlamydia, and possibly bacterial vaginosis organisms into the upper reproductive tract. Tubal occlusion prevents the egg from passing through the fallopian tubes.*

**Ectopic (tubal) pregnancy** *A potentially fatal condition that results when a fertilized egg implants outside the uterus, usually in the fallopian tubes. This type of pregnancy occurs when an ascending infection in the reproductive tract partially blocks tubal passages.*

**Genital cancers** *Potentially fatal diseases that have been associated with RTIs. Certain types of human papillomavirus (HPV) are associated with the development of cervical neoplasia.*

**Chronic pain** *May be experienced by patients with RTIs such as genital herpes and PID, which may cause persistent or episodic genital or abdominal pain.*

**Spectrum of HIV/AIDS symptoms** *Over the course of HIV infection, potentially the most serious RTI; the spectrum of symptoms includes acute retroviral illness, sore throat, swollen lymph nodes, increased skin rashes, herpes zoster, pulmonary tuberculosis, diarrhea, chronic fever, severe weight loss, bacterial pneumonia, invasive cancers, debilitating fatigue, simultaneous and recurrent infections, and, ultimately, death.*

*Adapted from: CDC. Family planning methods and practice: Africa. 2nd edition. Atlanta (GA): United States Department of Health and Human Services, CDC; 1999.*

awareness of the avoidability of adverse outcomes of pregnancy. Table 2 shows the proportion of pregnant women experiencing adverse outcomes by maternal diagnosis.

**Table 2. Proportion of Pregnant Women Experiencing Adverse Outcomes**

| Maternal Diagnosis | Fetal Wastage | Low Birth Weight or Prematurity | Congenital or Perinatal Infection |
|---|---|---|---|
| | % | % | % |
| Chlamydia | rare | 10–30 | 40–70 |
| Gonorrhea | rare | 11–25 | 30–68 |
| Early syphilis | 20–25 | 15–50 | 40–70 |
| Genital herpes | | | |
|     Primary | 7–54 | 30–50 | 30–35 |
|     Recurrent | rare | rare | 0.4–8 |
| Bacterial vaginosis | rare | 10–25 | rare |
| Trichomoniasis | rare | 11–15 | rare |
| No RTI | 4–10 | 2–12 | NA |

Adapted from: Wasserheit JN, Holmes KK. Reproductive tract infections: challenges for international health policy, programs, and research. In: Germain A, Holmes KK, Piot P, Wasserheit JN, editors. Reproductive tract infections: global impact and priorities for women's reproductive health. New York: Plenum Press; 1992. p. 16.

## How Are RTIs Transmitted?

RTIs are caused by bacterial, parasitic, and viral pathogens. Generally, the pathogens causing RTIs enter the body through the mucous membranes during unprotected vaginal, anal, or oral intercourse with an infected partner (5). An individual's risk of contracting an RTI or developing sequelae of an RTI is a function of five components: the risk of interaction with an infected person who may become a regular sex partner; exposure to the infection of that partner; acquisition of the RTI when exposed; development of a symptomatic RTI if infected; and development of the sequelae following the RTI (6). The same sexual behaviors may result in the acquisition of different RTIs, depending on which infections are most prevalent in a particular setting. Multiple infections within the same individual are also frequent, as is reinfection if partners have not been adequately treated.

For many STDs, the probability of transmission is higher from males to females than from females to males. Most STDs tend to exhibit a "biological sexism" (7); in other words, anatomic factors appear to make the transmission of STDs more efficient from male to female than from female to male. For example, the risk of acquiring gonorrhea from a single sex act (where one partner is infectious)

## Why do STDs affect women more severely than men?

Women are less able to prevent exposure to STDs than men largely because of the lack of female-controlled barrier methods and because women are often limited in their ability to negotiate the conditions under which intercourse occurs. Women are more likely than men to acquire STDs from a single sexual encounter since women have a larger surface area exposed during intercourse and longer contact time with pathogens compared with men. When transmission does occur, women are more likely than men to be asymptomatically infected and, as a consequence, are less likely to recognize symptoms and seek health care. Even when health care is sought, most STDs are more difficult to diagnose in women than in men. Furthermore, the potential for spread of infection to the upper genital tract (e.g., the uterus and fallopian tubes or the testicles) is greater in women than in men. Lastly, women tend to suffer more serious long-term consequences than men, including pelvic inflammatory disease, infertility, ectopic pregnancy, chronic pelvic pain, and cervical cancer.

is approximately 25% for men and 50% for women (7). Infections tend to occur at an earlier age in females and affect females more severely than men.

RTIs can also be transmitted from the mother to the fetus during pregnancy or to the newborn at delivery. Most adverse outcomes occur before birth or during the first 30 days after birth (8). Syphilis during pregnancy has been shown to cause infant death, adverse outcome, or syphilitic infants in more than 5% of cases where the pregnancy survives beyond 12 weeks. Gonococcal ophthalmia neonatorum occurs in 2%–6% of newborns. Table 3 shows the prevalence, rate of transmission from mother to child, and manifestations of selected RTIs.

## How Are RTIs and Their Sequelae Linked With Key Health-Related Development Programs?

A major challenge facing women with RTIs in developing countries is limited access to health care for those infections. Concepts of case management used in developed countries are usually inappropriate for implementation in developing countries in which care is provided through an array of services and individuals (3). In many parts of the world, women rely heavily on reproductive health services, particularly family planning and maternal/child health (FP/MCH) services, for most of their health needs. Other services attended by women include primary health care centers, general hospital outpatients, and private practice. A considerable amount of treatment for RTIs is offered by pharmacists, traditional healers, untrained lay people, and street vendors.

Most of the services attended by women in developing countries lack skilled personnel and access to the drugs required to detect and treat RTIs. The majority of clinics that are equipped to manage these infections primarily gear their services toward men. A response to these issues was the recommendation for the integration of prevention and treatment services for RTIs into other reproductive health services routinely attended by women, including family planning and prenatal clinics.

Serving women in the general population through existing health programs has become an essential part of RTI prevention and control. RTIs are an integral part of fundamental health-related development programs, such as these concerned with family planning, child survival, women's health, safe motherhood, and HIV prevention (see Figure 1, p. 10) (1).

**Table 3. Prevalence, Transmission Rates, and Manifestations of Selected RTIs**

| RTI | Prevalence of Infection in Pregnant Women | Fetal/Neonatal Transmission Rate | Incidence of the Manifestation Without Interventions |
|---|---|---|---|
| Adverse pregnancy outcomes caused by syphilis; *Treponema pallidum* | 0.03%–0.3% in industrialized countries; 3%–22% in Africa, parts of South America, and Fiji | Overall, 40%–70%; almost 100% if maternal syphilis is early stage; perhaps as low as 23% if late | At a seroprevalence of 10%, over 5% of all pregnant women would have an adverse outcome: 2% spontaneous abortions; 2.4% perinatal deaths; and 1.4% syphilitic infants. |
| Gonococcal ophthalmia neonatorum; *Neisseria gonorrhoeae* | Low: 1% or less, such as in Western Europe and some parts of North America High: 4%–20%, such as in sub-Saharan Africa and Thailand | 47%; 68% when concomitantly infected with *Chlamydia trachomatis* | 4%–6% of births in Africa; 2%–4% common in much of Africa. |
| Chlamydial ophthalmia neonatorum; *Chlamydia trachomatis* | Range: 2%–37% Common: 4%–12% Low: 0%–5% Medium: 6%–14% High: 15% and higher | Total: 60%–70% Conjunctivitis: 15%–50%; 15%–30% severe, 25% coming to medical care | Assuming a 10% seroprevalence, 2.5% of pregnancies would result in infants with conjunctivitis who are brought to medical care. |
| Chlamydial pneumonia; *Chlamydia trachomatis* | Range: 2%–37% Common: 4%–12% Low: 0%–5% Medium: 6%–14% High: 15% and higher | Pneumonia: 5%–15%; 5% coming to medical care | Assuming a 10% seroprevalence, 0.5% of pregnancies would result in infants with pneumonia. |
| Neonatal herpes; genital HSV | 20%–50% in the United States have developed antibodies to HSV; viral excretion at delivery is approximately 0.01%–0.39%; prevalence appears lower in other parts of the world | Primary infection: 50% Recurrent infection: 0.4%–8% | Incidence is 0.2%–0.33% per 1,000 live births in the United States, with overall mortality of 0.14%–0.23% per 1,000 live births. |
| HIV | | Industrialized countries: 15%–25% Developing countries: 25%–45% | |

Adapted from: Schulz KF, Schulte JM, Berman SM. Maternal health and child survival: opportunities to protect both women and children from the adverse consequences of reproductive tract infections. In: Germain A, Holmes KK, Piot P, Wasserheit JN, editors. Reproductive tract infections: global impact and priorities for women's reproductive health. New York: Plenum Press; 1992. p. 146.

Each of these health programs provides a critical opportunity for the prevention, detection, and control of RTIs with excellent opportunities to educate clients about modes of RTI transmission and prevention of future infection.

There can be serious limitations to integration, including an overemphasis on clinical management of STDs accompanied by significant problems in implementing clinical management protocols, as well as a lack of support for primary prevention, such as condom promotion and behavioral change interventions *(9)*.

A review that tried to clarify the public health benefits of integration found some evidence to suggest that where there was an emphasis on STD prevention, the quality of services, providers' attitudes, and communication skills improved *(10)*. However, there was inadequate evidence to show increased use of STD treatment services or an impact on STD rates. Because of these limitations of past efforts at integration, some guidelines have advocated for a focus on primary prevention (e.g., counseling and behavior change interventions, aggressive condom promotion, and social marketing) as well as prevention and treatment efforts targeted at "high transmitters," those most likely to contract and transmit STDs *(9)*.

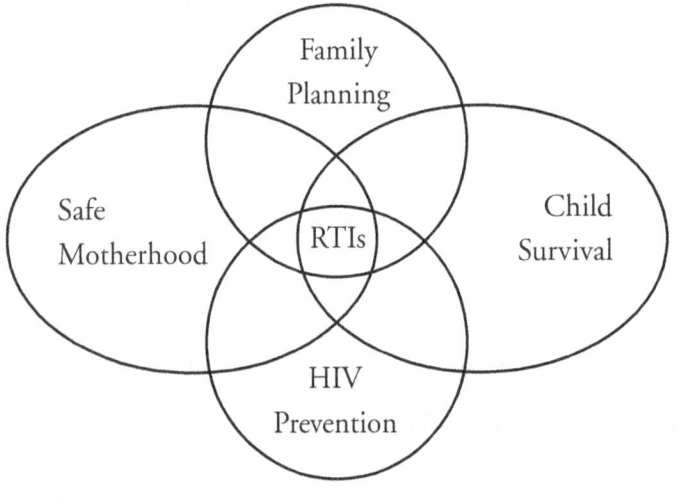

**Figure 1. The Role of RTIs in Health-Related Development Programs**

Source: Wasserheit JN, Holmes KK. Reproductive tract infections: challenges for international health policy, programs, and research. In: Germain A, Holmes KK, Piot P, Wasserheit JN, editors. Reproductive tract infections: global impact and priorities for women's reproductive health. New York: Plenum Press; 1992. p. 8.

Guidelines on when to integrate clinical STD or RTI management into FP/MCH programs highlight how epidemiology can be used to guide programmatic decisions *(9)*. (See "Integrating STD Clinical Services Into Family Planning and Maternal/Child Health Programs," p. 12.) The first steps are to determine the prevalence of various STDs in the FP/MCH population and to conduct drug sensitivity studies. These steps are critical in determining whether these services will have a public health benefit. The positive predictive value of any screening or diagnostic test will be higher in communities where the infection is more prevalent. The second step, assessing the risk profile of clientele who use the particular FP/MCH service delivery setting, can be done through risk assessment surveys of clients.

---

### Family Planning Services Provide an Opportunity to Treat Asymptomatic Genital Tract Infections in Rural South Africa

*A study was conducted among women attending the family planning clinic at Hlabisa Hospital, South Africa, to determine the prevalence of asymptomatic and unrecognized genital tract infections (11). As part of the study, women attending the family planning clinic were offered a gynecologic examination during which a vaginal swab and questionnaire were administered. Diagnostic testing of the swabs revealed that 119 (63%) of the 189 women had at least one infection and 49 (26%) had multiple infections. Of the 66 women with gonorrhea, chlamydial infection, trichomoniasis, or bacterial vaginosis, 35 (53%) were asymptomatic. Furthermore, many symptomatic women failed to recognize and report their symptoms. Results also revealed that 15 (8%) of the women had active syphilis and 44 (24%) tested positive for HIV. None of these cases were detected during routine family planning consultations, mainly because syphilis screening and HIV testing were not done by the family planning service, on-site microbiological facilities were unavailable, and many cases of infection were asymptomatic. Family planning providers in this setting could consider incorporating routine syphilis screening and HIV testing into existing services as a strategy to reduce the burden of RTIs in this setting.*

### Integrating STD Clinical Services Into Family Planning and Maternal/Child Health Programs

*B*efore integrating clinical STD services into FP/MCH programs, program managers should take the following minimum steps:

1. Determine the prevalence of various STDs in the FP/MCH population. Laboratory screening tests suitable for prevalence surveys are increasingly available and possess high sensitivity and specificity. The cost of these surveys is not excessive and sample sizes of 200–300 service delivery clients may be sufficient to guide decision making about locating and targeting integrated services. The prevalence of gonorrhea and chlamydia in typical FP/MCH settings in Africa is 6%–10%.

2. Assess the risk profile of clientele who use the FP/MCH service delivery setting. Integration of clinical STD services may be more justifiable in settings that serve a higher proportion of clients at high risk (e.g., commercial sex workers and their partners). Simple instruments can be used to determine basic demographic information and assess level of risk behavior.

3. Ascertain the level of staff expertise and available infrastructure.

4. Ensure that integrated FP/MCH interventions will receive necessary training, supervision, technical standards, and other organizational support to ensure that the quality of services delivered remains high.

5. Ensure that sufficient resources are available, especially for STD drugs, because STD drug procurement is not one of USAID's comparative advantages.

*Adapted from: USAID. Integration of family planning/MCH with HIV/STD prevention. Washington: USAID; December 1998.*

## GENERAL MODEL OF THE EPIDEMIOLOGY OF RTIs

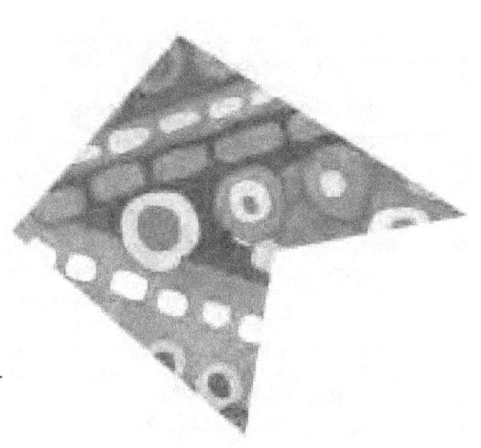

Epidemiology is used for measuring the distribution and determinants of health and illness in a population and for applying this information to the detection, prevention, and control of disease. Prevention and control of RTIs are made possible through surveillance and epidemiologic studies of disease etiology and transmission dynamics, treatment options, and intervention effectiveness. These studies help to explain the difference in risk of RTI among individuals within the same population and compare variations in the determinants of disease between populations *(12)*. Although biomedical research may explain why an exposure or behavior causes or prevents RTIs at the individual level, epidemiology adds to our understanding of the magnitude of the exposure/disease relationship in groups of individuals *(13)*. In some instances, such as HIV, epidemiologic research has provided information that has formed the basis for public health action long before the basic biologic mechanism of a particular disease was understood.

In some countries, epidemiologic studies provide information on the frequency of one or more RTIs in specific population groups. However, most of these studies are cross-sectional and provide information on the prevalence rather than the incidence of infection. Prevalence studies count all individuals within a population who have had the health problem at a specified point in time, regardless of the length of time the individuals have had the problem. In contrast, incidence studies aim to measure only the number of new cases of a health problem in a population within a specified period of time. One technique for estimating the actual magnitude of a health problem in a specific high-risk population is to exclude persons not at risk, since the overall incidence or prevalence rate may underrepresent the true extent of the disease in a particular subpopulation. For example, data for prevalence studies of STDs are often collected from a high-risk population, such as clients of STD clinics or commercial sex workers, and care should be taken in extrapolating from these studies to the general population *(14)*.

## How Is the Spread of RTIs Measured?

At the population level the rate of spread of STDs and RTIs is dependent on the average number of new cases generated by each infected individual. A number of biological characteristics of RTI pathogens influence the rate at which they spread and the usefulness of various control strategies *(15)*. The average rate of infectiousness also depends on the quality, accessibility, and uses of health services.

> **Transmission dynamics of STDs are approximated by**
>
> $$R_0 = \beta c D$$
>
> *where β is the average probability that the infection is transmitted per sexual partner contact per unit of time (efficiency of transmission), **c** is the average number of sexual partners per unit of time, and **D** is the average duration of infectiousness of an infected individual. The higher the value of **R**₀, the greater the potential for the spread of an STD. For an epidemic to occur,* $R_0 > 1$.

The average number of new cases generated by each infected individual is termed the basic reproductive rate of infection, or $R_0$. The basic reproductive infection rate is determined by the average probability that infection is transmitted from an infected individual to a susceptible individual ($\beta$), the effective mean rate of sexual partner change (c), and the average duration of infectivity (D).

The amount by which an infection's reproductive rate exceeds (or is below) 1.0 determines how rapidly the infection will spread (or be eliminated) in the community *(15)*. Although this measurement of reproductive success has many limitations, it is an important concept because the magnitude of reproductive success determines the pattern of infection and the rate at which an infection spreads when introduced into a susceptible population *(16)*. This model of STD transmission has been used to make predictions about epidemics and to specify factors that determine the rate of transmission or the process leading from initial infection to disease *(17)*.

## Efficiency of Transmission (β)

The efficiency of transmission ($\beta$) depends on the infectiousness of the pathogen, the infectivity of the infected individual, the susceptibility of the host, and the type of sexual act (e.g., vaginal, anal, or oral). For example, the use of barrier methods of contraception decreases the susceptibility of the host to infection, thereby decreasing the efficiency of transmission of many RTIs. Efficiency of transmission is also related to the size of the pathogen and is generally highest during early infection and when lesions or exudate are present. Other biological factors may also increase the risk that a susceptible person will acquire an RTI after exposure. For example, cervical ectopy (a process of squamous metaplasia that begins at menarche, in which the columnar epithelial cells around the cervical os are replaced by squamous epithelium) has been shown to increase the risk of chlamydial and gonorrheal infection *(2)*. Since cervical ectopy decreases as a woman ages and increases with oral contraceptive use, very young women and oral contraceptive users may be at higher risk of infection.

## Effective Mean Rate of Sexual Partner Change (c)

The basic reproductive infection rate in a population depends on the average number of sexual partners per person per unit of time, heterogeneity (differences) in rates of sexual partner change, patterns of sexual contact (i.e., who mixes with whom), and the types of contraceptives used and how they are used. In general, people with high rates of sexual partner change contribute disproportionately to the transmission of RTIs; however, rates of sexual partner change depend on many demographic and social factors.

# Duration of Infectiousness (D)

Early detection and treatment reduces the average length of time infected individuals are infectious and therefore reduces both the rate of spread of the infection as well as the probability that infected individuals will develop complications and sequelae *(2)*. The infectiousness of a particular individual is subject to great variation with respect to both duration and intensity *(16)*.

# How Is the Model of Transmission Dynamics Applied?

The variables in the transmission dynamics model can be translated into practical determinants of the spread of infection. For example, transmissibility of infection is influenced by behavioral factors such as the number of partners and susceptibility to infection is influenced by the use of barrier methods such as condoms. By clarifying demographic and social correlates of RTIs, women with increased risk of infection may be identified through routine screening, and measures can be taken to control and prevent the spread of infection in the population. Table 4 provides examples of biological, behavioral, medical, and social and economic factors affecting the spread of STDs and RTIs.

**Table 4. Factors Affecting the Spread of STDs and RTIs in a Population**

|  | Variable Affected |
|---|---|
| **Biological** | |
| Duration of infectivity | D |
| Presence of other STDs | $\beta$ |
| Infectivity of particular strain of the pathogen | $\beta$ |
| Age and presence of cervical erosion | $\beta$ |
| Immunologic status | $\beta$ |
| Circumcision status | $\beta$ |
| **Behavioral** | |
| Rates of sexual partner change | c |
| Type of sexual intercourse (anal, oral, vaginal) | $\beta$ |
| Use of condoms and other contraceptives | $\beta$, c |
| Patterns of sexual contact and mixing | c |
| **Medical** | |
| Access to health care facilities | D |
| Access to laboratory facilities | D |
| Availability of appropriate treatment | D |
| **Social and Economic** | |
| Migration patterns | c |
| Ease of travel | c |
| Level of education | c |
| Religion | c |
| Civil unrest | c |
| Position of women in society | c |

Adapted from: Rowley J, Berkley S. Sexually transmitted diseases. In: Murray CJL, Lopez AD, editors. Health dimensions of sex and reproduction. Boston: Harvard University Press; 1998. p. 27.

The basic reproductive rate of infection ($R_0$) model can be used as a tool for identifying the relative influences of different behavioral, biological, medical, and socioeconomic components on the rate at which different people acquire infection and has implications for the design and implementation of control and prevention programs. For example, infections that are transmitted more efficiently may contribute to rapid increases in the incidence of RTIs through the activities of potential high-frequency transmitters such as prostitutes (15). In these cases, control efforts that reduce transmission by core group members may rapidly affect the incidence of those RTIs.

# LONG-TERM OUTCOME INDICATORS FOR STDs AND RTIs

Indicators are measurements that, when compared with either a standard or desired level of achievement, provide information regarding a health outcome of a management process. Useful indicators serve as markers of progress toward improved reproductive health status, either as a direct or proxy measure of impact (outcome indicator), or as a measure of progress toward specified process goals (process indicator) *(18)*. This discussion will focus on outcome measures that reflect changes in mortality, morbidity, and other health outcomes.

Conceptually, the long-term goal of RTI control and prevention programs is improved reproductive health at the population level, but it is often difficult to link changes in long-term indicators directly to a particular intervention program. For this reason, many evaluations are limited to simply monitoring change in key indicators over time *(19)*. Researchers interested in using indicators to evaluate specific programs should choose those most relevant to the objectives of the program. The following indicators provide examples of types of measures useful in monitoring progress toward reduction of HIV, STDs, and RTIs *(19)*:

## RTI Prevalence in a Defined Target Population

*Definition.* This measure is defined as the number of persons diagnosed with a specific RTI or syndrome at a given point in time per 100,000 persons in the population (or population sub-group, defined by such characteristics as age, gender, and place of residence) and is calculated as follows:

$$\frac{\text{Number of RTIs identified by syndromic signs/symptoms or etiologic (serologic/culture) methods}}{\text{Number of people in population group screened or covered by case reports}} \times 100{,}000$$

Data sources for the numerator include special laboratory-based surveys, sentinel surveillance, and case (syndromic or etiologic) and laboratory reports from clinicians and diagnostic laboratories. When the numerator is found through special laboratory-based surveys or sentinel surveillance, the denominator is the number of people screened. If the numerator is the number of case and laboratory reports from clinicians and diagnostic laboratories, the denominator is the number of people in the population (or population subgroup) served by the reporting facilities.

***Use and Interpretation.*** It is important to emphasize that this is a measure of prevalence rather than incidence and provides an estimate of the current situation regarding RTIs in the sample population for the period of testing. In some settings, however, this indicator can resemble a measure of incidence. For example, in Sweden the level of gonorrhea has been controlled for nearly 30 years. In this setting it is highly likely that any cases reported in a recent calendar year would be new cases; thus, the calculation of prevalence may approximate the incidence rate of gonorrhea. The use of cross-sectional surveys to determine the prevalence of RTIs is generally considered the best method since it is possible to define the population at risk by controlling the sampling frame, and to avoid many of the biases inherent to other methods (for example, sentinel surveillance and case reporting methods); however, this method requires considerable infrastructure (laboratory and statistical) and resources.

## Infertility

***Definition.*** This measure is defined as the proportion of sexually active noncontracepting women in a reproductive age group (usually 15–45 years) at risk of pregnancy who have not had any pregnancies in the previous 5 years and is calculated as follows:

$$\frac{\text{Number of women in the specified age group who are not using contraceptives (and have not done so in the past 5 years), are not pregnant, and have not had a child in the last 5 years}}{\text{Total number of women in the specified age group who are at risk of pregnancy (i.e., those who are not using contraceptives, and are not pregnant)}} \times 100{,}000$$

Data sources for estimating infertility include the Demographic Health Survey data and fertility surveys.

***Use and Interpretation.*** This indicator measures the level of infertility in a community. A level of 5% or less is to be expected in all populations because of inherent reproductive abnormalities. The most common cause of increased rates of tubal infertility in many countries is STDs. For example, the proportion of infertility attributable to RTIs is 50%–80% in Africa, 15%–40% in Asia, 35% in

Latin America, and 10%–35% in industrialized countries *(1)*. Therefore, to some extent this indicator is a measure of consequence of STD in a community. The period of 5 years is a generous time interval since it is generally accepted that 90% of all couples will achieve pregnancy within 2 years if they have regular intercourse and do not use contraception.

## STD/HIV-Related Cause-Specific Mortality Rate

*Definition.* This indicator combines four life-threatening diagnoses related to STD/HIV into one measure of mortality. It is an estimate of the STD/HIV-related cause-specific death rate among women of reproductive age due to four leading causes: AIDS; cervical cancer due to HPV; PID; and ectopic pregnancy. This indicator is calculated as follows:

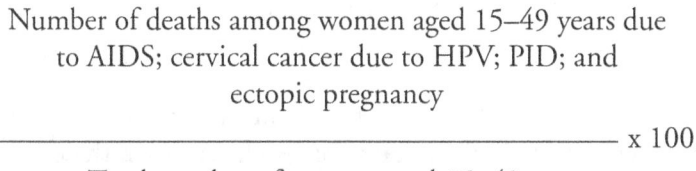

$$\frac{\text{Number of deaths among women aged 15–49 years due to AIDS; cervical cancer due to HPV; PID; and ectopic pregnancy}}{\text{Total number of women aged 15–49 years}} \times 100{,}000$$

The data source for this measure is hospital records indicating cause-specific mortality among women of reproductive age.

*Use and Interpretation.* This measure underscores the idea that the long-term goal of STD/HIV intervention programs is to lower mortality by reducing the risk of exposure to infection. However, programs are not usually evaluated by this measure because it is virtually impossible to separate the effects of program intervention from other external factors (such as socioeconomic conditions) on this outcome. Furthermore, behavioral changes leading to reductions in STD/HIV incidence will require several years to have a noticeable impact on this mortality rate.

Prevalence rates of these four diseases may vary across countries, and those diagnoses that are most life-threatening in a region should be given special consideration. Also, the ability to diagnose certain infections may vary depending on the medical technology available in a region, or whether etiologic testing or the syndromic approach is used to detect infections. The mortality rate may appear to increase in areas in which screening services are improved because of better case detection. This indicator may be adapted to specific age groups (e.g., 15–24, 25–34, 35 years and older) to enhance its cultural or geographical relevance.

# Rate of Congenital Syphilis or Ophthalmia Neonatorum

*Definition.* This indicator is the number of infants born infected with syphilis or with gonococcal/chlamydial eye infections during a specific time period (usually one year) per 100,000 live births. This indicator is calculated as follows:

$$\frac{\text{Number of cases of infants born with congenital syphilis (CS) or ophthalmia neonatorum (ON)}}{\text{Number of live births among population covered by case reports}} \times 100{,}000$$

The data sources for the numerator include case and laboratory reports from clinicians, clinical settings, and diagnostic laboratories. Vital records serve as the data source for the denominator.

*Use and Interpretation.* Theoretically this measure could be used as a marker of STD at the population level. However, there are significant diagnostic problems associated with case definition of CS and ON, especially in resource-poor settings. The appropriate diagnostics may not be universally applied to all births, resulting in underdetection of cases. For congenital syphilis, the most appropriate diagnostics relate to the mother. Syphilis prevalence data for pregnant women provide information about both latent and symptomatic syphilis in this group and minimize the problems associated with general reporting of RTIs. Because the primary lesion is often painless and secondary syphilis is usually not diagnosed, women are mainly identified through serological screening. As with all case reporting systems, the quality of the data is influenced by the providers who make the diagnosis and the system of health statistics and infrastructure.

# SURVEILLANCE FOR RTIS

Surveillance is an essential component of effective prevention and control programs for RTIs and is used to determine the need for public health action and assess the effectiveness of interventions and programs. Surveillance is an important means of obtaining baseline information before establishing RTI services. It is also a mechanism for collecting the information needed to calculate the long-term indicators discussed earlier. Ongoing surveillance is used to identify temporal trends in RTI morbidity and is often used to guide decisions regarding the allocation of resources for control and prevention programs.

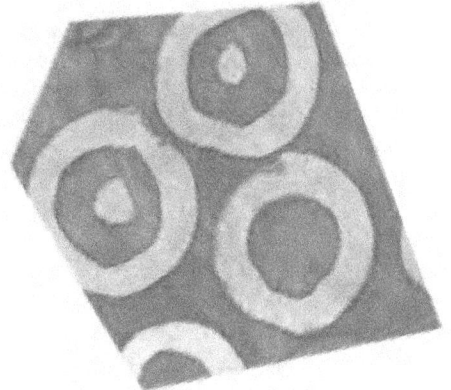

### Surveillance for STDs in the Russian Federation

A state system for the control and surveillance of STDs in which diagnosis, treatment, and partner notification are provided by clinical Dermatovenereology Service dispensaries has existed in the Russian Federation since World War II (20). In 1993, the notification by physicians of newly identified cases of nine STDs (syphilis, gonorrhea, trichomoniasis, urogenital chlamydiosis, human papillomavirus infection, genital herpes, mycoplasmosis, candidiasis, and bacterial vaginosis) was mandated. Through this system of surveillance, researchers noticed a 63-fold increase in the rate of syphilis from 1993 to 1997. Although improvements in laboratory techniques for diagnosis have been suggested as the reason for this apparent increase, it is also likely that the cause is related to the economic and political changes occurring in the Russian Federation. Shifts in living standards, working conditions, health services funding, and migration rates, and changes in social infrastructure following the breakup of the Soviet Union are factors that may affect the occurrence of syphilis. Of particular concern is the high rate of syphilitic morbidity among children and adolescents—26,000 cases were reported in 1997. These population-based findings are especially relevant for public health officials, who must base their control and prevention strategies on estimates of the burden of STDs and their distribution within the population.

Reporting cases may be mandatory or voluntary, but ideally every country should have an active RTI surveillance system to which cases of disease are reported. In countries that have good vital registration and reporting systems, the number of reported cases is a reliable proxy for the total number of infections of disease with very definite symptoms (2). Sources of information include medical records, health care facilities, commercial and reference laboratories, and research projects. In general, specialty STD clinics tend to be the most reliable at reporting cases of infection, followed by government facilities and, lastly, private practitioners (2).

Rapid assessment is another important method for collecting data that uses a similar methodology and is fraught with many of the same issues as surveillance. Unlike surveillance, which is ongoing, rapid assessment is an accelerated form of epidemiologic research used to determine the prevalence of a condition at a point in time and rapidly link the information to public health action. In some situations this method is preferable to conventional epidemiologic research approaches, which can be time-consuming and often lack the capacity to inform policy or program decision making in time. Rapid assessment may be especially important in acute emergency or crisis situations where timely interventions are necessary to improve the reproductive health of women.

---

**Performing a Rapid Assessment for STDs in a Rwandan Refugee Camp in Tanzania**

*In the aftermath of the genocide of Rwanda in 1994, more than 300,000 people crossed the border with Tanzania within a few weeks and were confined in two camps in northwest Tanzania. The disintegrating social structure was conducive to the transmission of STDs and HIV. During the initial phase of the refugee camps, there was little data on the prevalence of STDs. Information was needed to target STD service delivery more efficiently (21).*

*In a weeklong rapid assessment, 100 women attending one antenatal clinic were given a full physical and gynecological examination, during which vaginal swabs were collected for immediate wet preparation and gram staining, cervical swabs were collected for Neisseria gonorrhoeae (NG) culture, and blood samples were collected for syphilis serology. STD indicators were validated against a confirmatory laboratory test indicating the presence or absence of STD. All patients found to have a vaginal discharge were treated upon first visit. Results of syphilis serology were communicated privately, and treatment was provided 2 weeks after the initial visit.*

*Results of the rapid assessment revealed that the prevalence of RTIs in these women was 60%, if candidiasis and bacterial vaginosis were included. It was also found that 60% of women who had an abnormal vaginal discharge upon examination actually reported a symptom related to genital discharge syndrome (discharge, genital itching, lower abdominal pain, dysuria, or dyspareunia), showing a good correlation between reported symptoms and confirmed signs. Women should be encouraged by clinic staff to report genital symptoms. Etiological diagnosis solely by type of discharge is not recommended— for example, all three women infected with NG were also infected by Trichomonas vaginalis, so symptoms for each infection could not be separated. It is important that all health-delivery staff be aware of how to recognize STDs in emergency settings. Rapid STD assessment can be useful in obtaining quick and reliable information at a relatively low cost. In this situation, results of the assessment provided a basis for case projection and budget planning. A second rapid assessment will be conducted later to evaluate the impact of these changes.*

Surveillance and rapid assessment surveys are useful tools for obtaining information to guide public health efforts to reduce morbidity and mortality associated with RTIs. Determining the level of morbidity in a population has important implications for influencing STD/RTI program activity *(22)*. Three epidemiologic measures of disease frequency are commonly used: case counts, proportions, and incidence. These measures are useful for calculating the long-term outcome indicators discussed earlier. For accuracy of all measures of disease frequency, care must be taken in distinguishing between incident, prevalent, and recurrent infections.

---

### Important Definitions in Measuring Disease Frequency

*Incidence of disease* The number of new cases of the disease of interest occurring in a population during a defined time interval.

*Prevalence of disease* The proportion of people in a population who have the disease of interest at a specified point in time.

*Recurrence of disease* Diagnosis of the disease of interest after receiving adequate treatment for this same disease.

---

*Case Counts.* Perhaps the simplest way of reporting morbidity is to report the number of cases identified by counting the number of new (incident) or existing (prevalent) cases of the disease in the population during a given period of time. However, a count does not provide any information about the size of the population in which the cases were identified and, thus, is often referred to as "numerator" data. Counts may be valuable in a particular population for allocating limited resources. For example, a large number of cases of a particular RTI identified in the community may require program personnel to direct program resources toward treating those cases and preventing spread of infection to others in the community.

*Proportions.* A proportion is defined as a fraction in which the numerator is included in the denominator. The numerator of a proportion is generated through case counts. Some previously described measures, such as the STD/HIV-related cause-specific mortality rate and the rate of congenital syphilis, are examples of proportions. A proportion at a particular point in time is often expressed as a percentage (for example, clients who are appropriately managed for RTIs in a given month divided by all clients seen in that month).

Proportions are used in a wide range of public health activities. For example, if a large proportion of the reproductive morbidity in a community is associated with a particular RTI, program personnel may decide to concentrate outreach activities, expand clinic facilities, or work with community-based organizations in that area to reduce the burden of morbidity in the community due to that infection. In terms of RTI prevention and control, prevalence is a proportion that measures how widespread an infection is in a population, the amount of infection that needs to be treated in a population, and how much of that population may experience adverse sequelae if the disease is untreated or not treated in a timely manner.

*Incidence Rates.* An incidence rate is a measure of risk and the most common way of measuring frequency of disease in populations. This measure is a fraction in which the numerator is the number of people that develop a disease during a given time period (new cases), and the denominator is the population *at risk* for the disease during the same time period. (Note that in settings with stable prevalence of infection, it is likely that any cases reported in a recent calendar year would be new cases; thus, the calculation of prevalence may actually approximate the incidence rate.) Incidence rates are useful for comparing the risk of disease between populations because they relate the number of new cases in each community to a population base. For many RTIs and STDs, the population at risk (denominator) would include only those people who are sexually active, a subgroup that is often difficult to identify. Obtaining accurate numerator and denominator data can be quite challenging but is an essential part of increasing awareness about the magnitude, sequelae, and preventability of RTIs.

An accurate assessment of the dimensions of a problem enables policy and decision makers to focus their attention and resources on measures to control and prevent the spread of disease. WHO has developed comprehensive guidelines for the surveillance of STDs that can be accessed at the following Web site: http://www.who.int/emc-documents/STIs/docs/STI%20Guidelines.html (Note: a synonymous term for STDs used by WHO is sexually transmitted infections or STIs). The Centers for Disease Control and Prevention (CDC) has developed guidelines for evaluating surveillance systems that can be accessed at the following Web site: http://www.cdc.gov/mmwr/preview/mmwrhtml/rr5013a1.htm. For more detail on designing and implementing reproductive health surveillance systems, and analysis of surveillance data, see the *Reproductive Health Surveillance Module.*

## What Are Some Issues in Surveillance of RTIs?

Even good surveillance systems vary greatly in their accuracy and completeness, and many RTIs are asymptomatic or have non-specific symptoms, making case diagnosis and reporting difficult. Self-treatment using medications from pharmacists and use of traditional remedies are common in many parts of the world. As a result, many infected women do not visit health clinics, and those who do seek care may be improperly diagnosed or not treated. The collection of data on RTIs is made more difficult because the highest prevalence of RTIs is often found within socially marginalized or stigmatized groups, such as prostitutes and substance abusers, or groups that are relatively inaccessible to health care providers and researchers, such as adolescents *(13)*. The social stigma associated with RTIs may deter women from attending STD clinics and result in women seeking care from alternative providers who may be less likely to report cases. Accordingly, not all cases are reported and the total number of new cases for many RTIs is often underestimated. In addition, reliable data on the complications and sequelae of RTIs, such as pelvic inflammatory disease and ectopic pregnancy, are few, even though complications are the cause of much of the burden of morbidity associated with RTIs.

## Laboratory-Based Surveillance

The traditional approach to the diagnosis and treatment of RTIs is through laboratory diagnosis to determine the etiologic agent causing infection. Laboratory tests are used to confirm symptomatic infections, to detect asymptomatic infections, to perform epidemiologic surveillance, and to monitor disease sensitivity to antibiotic treatment (antibiotic resistance). Ideally, laboratory tests for specific RTIs should be simple to perform, sensitive and specific, rapid, inexpensive, and should not require special equipment. Two important concepts in laboratory-based RTI surveillance are *sensitivity* and *specificity* (Appendix B). Sensitivity indicates how accurately a test can identify diseased persons and specificity indicates how accurately a test can identify those who are free of disease.

Although the use of laboratory diagnostics is the preferred approach, it tends to be expensive in terms of tests, equipment, and laboratory maintenance and often results in delays in diagnosis and treatment. In reality, simple, affordable, and accurate diagnostic tests are not currently available for many RTIs. In many developing regions, it is usually not possible to detect the pathogen since most clinics lack the capacity, resources, training, or laboratory support to comprehensively examine clients for RTIs *(5)*.

## Is There an Alternative to Laboratory-Based Surveillance in Resource-Poor Settings?

In response to the limitations of laboratory-based surveillance in many parts of the world, WHO developed a syndromic approach to RTI management. The syndromic approach to RTI management uses clinical algorithms based on STD syndromes (i.e., the pattern of patient symptoms and clinical signs) to determine antimicrobial therapy *(23)*. Using this approach, groups of symptoms and signs of infection are identified without laboratory tests and treatment is administered for all possible infections using drugs of proven local efficacy.

> *Syndromic diagnosis* is based on identifying consistent groups of symptoms and easily recognized signs, or syndromes, and providing treatment that will deal with the majority of organisms responsible for producing each syndrome.
>
> Source: World Health Organization. Guidelines for the management of sexually transmitted infections. Geneva, Switzerland: World Health Organization; 2001.

The syndromic approach can be used with minimal economic resources and is currently implemented in primary health centers in several parts of the world. The advantages of this approach include treatment at first visit, expedited care, cost savings because expensive laboratory tests are not used, and increased client satisfaction *(23)*. Providing treatment at the first visit reduces the risk of losing patients and having no follow-up care, and this in turn reduces further transmission and complications from untreated infections. The use of flowcharts in RTI management can help to standardize the diagnosis, treatment, referral, and reporting of STDs, which allows for improved surveillance and program management. However, the syndromic approach has many limitations that must be recognized, including the large number of asymptomatic infections, the lack of sensitivity and specificity for some diagnoses, and the variability in the performance of the decision models based on the clinical skills of the provider *(23)*.

A variety of demographic, behavioral, and clinical factors can also be used to assess the likelihood that a woman is currently infected with an RTI or is at high risk of future infection *(24)*. These factors can then be used to guide the syndromic management of infections in symptomatic patients (especially among women with vaginal discharge) and to identify asymptomatic clients who might need further clinical examination or laboratory evaluation *(25)*.

A review of several studies that evaluated the effectiveness of various syndromic management algorithms, including risk assessments, concluded that algorithms for urethral discharge and genital ulcer disease can be effective in detecting those infections, given their relatively high sensitivities and specificities *(26)*. However, the sensitivities and specificities for the vaginal discharge algorithms varied considerably from one study to another and overall were not found to be effective in detecting vaginal infections, particularly among asymptomatic or low-risk women.

## Issues in Monitoring Progress Toward the Reduction of RTIs

Estimating the magnitude of the morbidity associated with RTIs is a challenging task; nevertheless, determining the magnitude of the problem is essential so that progress toward the reduction of RTIs may be monitored. Self-reporting of RTIs in women is unreliable because of nonrecognition of symptoms and the high rate of asymptomatic infections *(18)*. Sentinel surveillance and case reporting methods are highly sensitive to site selection, use or provision of services, health infrastructure, and provider compliance in reporting. The ability to diagnose certain infections may vary depending on medical technology available. As screening services improve, rates of RTIs may appear higher because of better case detection. For these reasons, the validity, reliability, and representativeness of estimates are widely variable and should be regarded with caution; nevertheless, surveillance should be considered an essential part of monitoring RTIs to determine the need for public health action and to evaluate the effectiveness of RTI prevention and control programs.

## GENERAL MODEL AS FRAMEWORK FOR STRATEGIC PLANNING FOR CONTROL AND PREVENTION OF RTIs

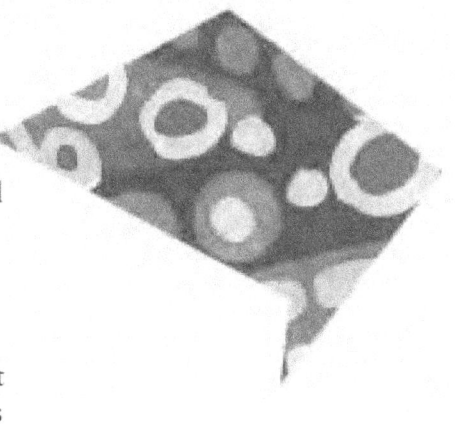

Although strategies for RTI control programs vary between developed and developing countries and within countries, the two basic principles that are common to all programs are 1) the prevention of the development of RTIs, their complications, and sequelae; and 2) the interruption and reduction of the transmission of RTIs (3). Effective control programs encourage the avoidance of behaviors likely to result in disease acquisition and transmission and ensure optimal treatments for RTIs. In individuals, early and effective treatment of RTIs is considered an essential component of the control of RTIs and HIV. At the population level, early and effective treatment prevents further transmission of RTIs and reduces HIV transmission (23). Identifying infected individuals, both symptomatic and asymptomatic, also plays an important role in control programs. Infected people can be detected through screening of those at high risk for RTI, through syndromic diagnosis and treatment, and by increasing the availability and rapidity of treatment, thus improving partner tracking and notification. Occasionally, identification of individuals is bypassed with mass treatment to eradicate the pathogen in a core group identified as having a high prevalence of RTI.

---

### General Principles for RTI Control

*The main goals of RTI control are accomplished by the following steps:*

1. *Reducing exposure to infection by educating people at risk to reduce the number of sex partners and to avoid sexual intercourse with people who have a high probability of being infected.*

2. *Preventing infection by promoting the use of condoms or other prophylactic barriers.*

3. *Detecting and curing disease by implementing disease detection activities, providing adequate diagnostic and treatment facilities, and promoting health-seeking behavior.*

4. *Limiting complications and further transmission of infection by providing early and appropriate treatment for symptomatic and asymptomatic patients and their sex partners, and through counseling.*

*Adapted from: Meheus A, Schulz K, Cates W. Development of prevention and control programs for sexually transmitted diseases in developing countries. In: Holmes KK, Mardh P, Sparling PF, Wiesner PJ, Cates W, Lemon SM, et al., editors. Sexually transmitted disease. New York: McGraw-Hill; 1990. p. 1041–6.*

Most bacterial and parasitic genital infections are fully curable with antibiotics. Disease control strategies based on early diagnosis and treatment and health-seeking behaviors are important determinants of the incidence of curable RTIs (27). However, not all curable RTIs can be controlled equally. This is especially true in developing countries, where the absence of resources necessary for diagnosis makes certain curable infections (e.g., gonorrheal or chlamydial infection) comparable to the incurable viral RTIs.

Although viral infections cannot currently be cured, their complications may be minimized. For this reason, health-seeking behaviors are still important in the epidemiology of these diseases. However, primary prevention remains the key intervention. Control strategies for viral RTIs largely depend on efforts at primary prevention through health education of the community and individualized counseling of infected carriers (27). For example, HIV can be transmitted from an infected woman to her fetus or newborn during pregnancy, during labor and delivery, and during the postpartum period (through breastfeeding). Perinatal transmission rates ranging from 13% to 40% have been estimated, depending on the prevalence of various factors that influence the likelihood of HIV transmission. For this reason, HIV counseling and testing for women of childbearing age offer important prevention opportunities for both uninfected (primary prevention) and infected (secondary prevention) women and their infants.

Comprehensive guidelines for the treatment of patients who have STDs were developed by CDC and can be accessed at: http://www.cdc.gov/std/treatment/TOC2002TG.htm.

## Prevention of RTIs

Although some RTIs are not curable, all are preventable. Generally speaking, primary prevention activities are designed to reduce the occurrence of disease before the pathogen has interacted with the host (28). Secondary prevention occurs after the pathogens have interacted with the host, and intends to reduce the progression of the disease.

Prevention of RTIs is an important message for all people, including those at low risk. Primary prevention involves avoiding infection in the first place; the most effective way to prevent sexual transmission of RTIs is to avoid sexual intercourse with infected partners. Secondary prevention reduces the likelihood of complications and sequelae of RTIs. Prevention goals require that people adopt preventive behaviors (such as avoiding unprotected intercourse with infected partners) and

**General Guidelines for the Prevention of RTIs/STDs**

*The best way to prevent sexually transmitted diseases (STDs) and reproductive tract infections (RTIs) is to not have sexual relations. However, if you do decide to be sexually active, there are ways to reduce the risk of contracting an STD or RTI:*

- *Ask a new sex partner if he or she has an STD/RTI, has been exposed to one, or has any unexplained physical symptoms. Do not have sex if your partner has signs or symptoms, such as sores, rashes, or discharge from the genital area.*

- *Many common STDs/RTIs have no symptoms but can still be transmitted to a sexual partner. If your partner has had sexual relations with someone else recently, they may have an infection, even if there are no symptoms. Therefore, do not have sex if you think your partner may have been exposed to an STD/ RTI, even if they do not show any symptoms.*

- *Use a condom correctly and consistently during all types of sexual intercourse (oral, vaginal, and anal).*

- *Get regular checkups for STDs and RTIs (even if you show no symptoms), and be familiar with the common symptoms.*

- *Most bacterial infections are readily treated, and the earlier treatment is sought and sex partners are warned, the less likely the disease will do irreparable damage.*

*Source: CDC National Prevention Information Network (NPIN) Web site (www.cdcnpin.org/scripts/std/ index.asp).*

that clinicians diagnose and treat existing infections effectively *(7)*. Especially since the advent of the AIDS epidemic, initiatives to market and encourage the use of condoms have been central to RTI control programs because condoms reduce acquisition and transmission of both RTIs and HIV infection *(29)*.

## How Do Strategies for the Control and Prevention of Viral and Bacterial RTIs Differ?

There are significant differences in incidence, trends, distribution, and epidemiologic determinants between incurable, viral RTIs and curable, mostly bacterial RTIs. Health-seeking behaviors and disease control strategies based on early diagnosis and treatment are important determinants of the incidence of the curable RTIs. The traditional interventions of secondary prevention and management applied to bacterial RTIs will have a threefold effect: 1) to decrease transmission of bacterial RTIs within communities; 2) to reduce the reproductive sequelae of those RTIs; and 3) to slow the HIV epidemic, particularly through controlling genital ulcers.

Health-seeking behaviors are less effective in the epidemiology of incurable, viral RTIs. Mainly due to the increasing importance of incurable, viral RTIs, particularly HIV, strategies for primary prevention are receiving much higher priority today than in the past decade *(28)*. The epidemiologic synergy between HIV and other RTIs is an important concept underlying RTI risk *(7)*. Strong evidence indicates that both ulcerative and nonulcerative RTIs significantly increase the risk of acquiring and subsequently transmitting HIV. Preexisting STDs, such as herpes simplex virus, syphilis, and chancroid, especially when associated with genital tract ulcers, increase women's vulnerability to the transmission of HIV three to five times *(30)*. Furthermore, because the impaired immune system caused by HIV disease leads to persistent ulcerative symptoms, the infections have a direct effect on each other. Infections characterized by vaginal or urethral discharge (e.g., gonorrhea and chlamydia) have also been associated with higher levels of HIV infection. Because these infections are more common than genital ulcers, they make up a larger proportion of HIV transmission. Primary prevention efforts to reduce risky sexual behavior will not only help reduce the risk of HIV, but will be beneficial in the prevention of all RTIs. RTI control activities reduce the likelihood of transmission to sex partners; thus prevention for individuals translates into prevention for the community *(29)*.

# IMPLICATIONS OF RESEARCH AND USES OF COLLECTED DATA

Surveillance systems and descriptive epidemiologic studies show the frequency, distribution, and trends of disease within populations and are used to detect changes that may necessitate control measures or further research. Analytical studies provide measures of the strength of the association between particular characteristics, behaviors, exposures, or interventions, and the occurrence of disease.

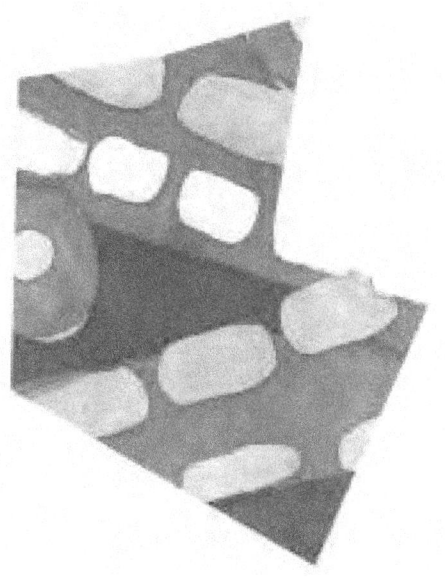

## How Are Surveillance Data Used?

Data from both surveillance systems and epidemiologic studies play an important role in informing the design, implementation, and evaluation of RTI treatment and prevention programs. These data may be used for setting public health priorities, planning, resource allocation, and identifying population subgroups and risky behaviors for targeted interventions *(13)*.

Epidemiologic data are particularly important in settings with limited resources for establishing priorities and guiding decision making. In these settings, cost-effectiveness studies of RTI control programs are especially important as a means of securing the necessary resources.

In all settings, epidemiologic data can provide useful information for diagnostic and therapeutic practice and indicate areas for further research. Epidemiologic studies can pave the way for the development of indicators and practical ways of estimating the burden of RTIs at the local level; laboratory-based surveillance can provide information on antimicrobial susceptibilities of infectious agents *(31)*. The challenge for those involved in surveillance or epidemiologic studies is to present their data in ways that will initiate effective control measures and to ensure that control programs are data-driven *(13)*.

## Who Needs to Know the Results of the Research, and Why?

Interpreting and communicating the results are the next steps in the process of transforming the data into information for action. Good data play a crucial role in allowing health staff to modify and refine field operations and also in focusing the attention of policymakers on the burden of morbidity and mortality due to RTIs. Therefore, those who need to know the findings include those who are the source of the primary data (such as health care providers and laboratory personnel) as well as those who are involved in administrative, program planning, and decision-making activities.

Results and recommendations serve to inform and motivate health personnel who are more likely to continue the challenging job of collecting information if they know that the information is being used and acted on. Feedback is important between the regional and national levels. For example, a need may be identified for training or resources at the local level that can only be obtained from the regional level. This communication may be facilitated through periodic meetings at the regional and national levels.

## How Can We Tell Whether an RTI Control Program Is Achieving Its Goals?

To assess the degree to which a control program is achieving its goals and targets, a system for monitoring and evaluation must be feasible. Regular review of RTI control and prevention programs allows health staff to modify and refine health actions taking place in the field. Evaluation is an important step in promoting the best use of public health resources and should include recommendations for improving quality and efficiency. Most importantly, an evaluation should assess whether the program is serving a useful public health function and is meeting its overall objective of reducing the burden of morbidity and mortality due to RTIs.

Evaluation generally involves the definition of indicators to track the program's progress toward explicit objectives. Once the objectives of a program have been defined, indicators (such as the long-term outcome indicators discussed earlier) are used as markers of progress toward those objectives. An indicator can be thought of as a measurement that provides information regarding a health outcome compared with a standard or desired level of achievement. The calculation of these indicators can be repeated over time as a measure of progress. For example, repeated measurement of an indicator, such as the prevalence of RTIs in a defined target population, is integral in the evaluation of the effectiveness and impact of a program aimed at improving reproductive health or achieving specific targets (e.g., a reduction in maternal morbidity).

In summary, the goal of evaluation is to:

- Select appropriate interventions that reflect local needs.

- Build on lessons learned and programs that have worked in other countries.

- Implement interventions according to current best practices.

- Monitor progress.

Evaluation can be used to guide the planning of effective RTI control and prevention programs, improve existing programs, and demonstrate the results of resource investments and interventions such as large-scale integration of services.

Reproductive tract infections continue to be a major and growing public health issue in many parts of the world and are particularly widespread in resource-poor settings. Without early diagnosis and appropriate therapy, complications of RTIs severely compromise women's health, fertility, and productivity; infant health and survival; and the effectiveness of family planning programs. Interventions that truly decrease the burden of RTIs will involve the coordination of efforts among several interrelated health initiatives and will include changes in the outlook, knowledge, skills, and resources of all levels of the health care system.

# RESOURCES

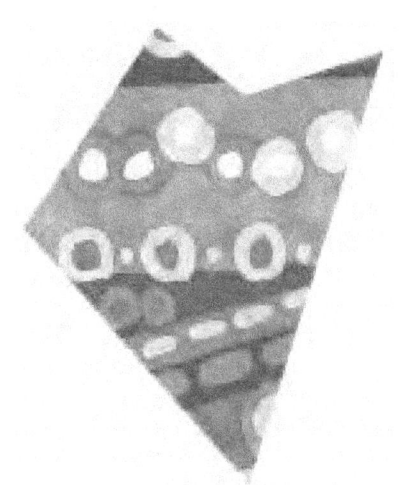

Selected RTI/STD/HIV Information Web sites (Adapted from: Hatcher RA, Trussell J, Stewart F, Cates W, Stewart GK, Guest F, et al. Contraceptive technology. New York: Ardent Media; 1998. p. 273–4.)

**AIDS Research and Information:**
http://www.CritPath.Org/aric

**AIDSCAP:**
http://www.fhi.org/en/aids/aidscap/aidsinfo/aidsinfo.html

**American Social Health Association:**
http://www.ashastd.org

**Association François-Xavier Bagnoud:**
http://www.fxb.org/indexeng.html

**Centers for Disease Control and Prevention:**
http://www.cdc.gov/nchstp/dstd/dstdp.html

**CDC National Prevention Information Network:**
http://www.cdcnpin.org

**Harvard University School of Public Health:**
http://www.hsph.harvard.edu

**HIVNET:**
http://www.hivnet.ch/e/index-frame.html

**Institute Pasteur:**
http://www.pasteur.fr/english.html

**International AIDS Society:**
http://www.ias.se

**National Center for HIV, STD & TB Prevention:**
http://www.cdc.gov/nchstp/od/nchstp.html

**National Institute of Allergy and Infectious Diseases (NIAID):**
http://www.niaid.nih.gov

**Population Services International (PSI):**
http://www.psi.org

**Tulane University AIDS Database:**
http://www.tulane.edu/~aids_db/database.htm

# CASE STUDY I

## EPIDEMIOLOGY OF STDS: OUTBREAK INVESTIGATION

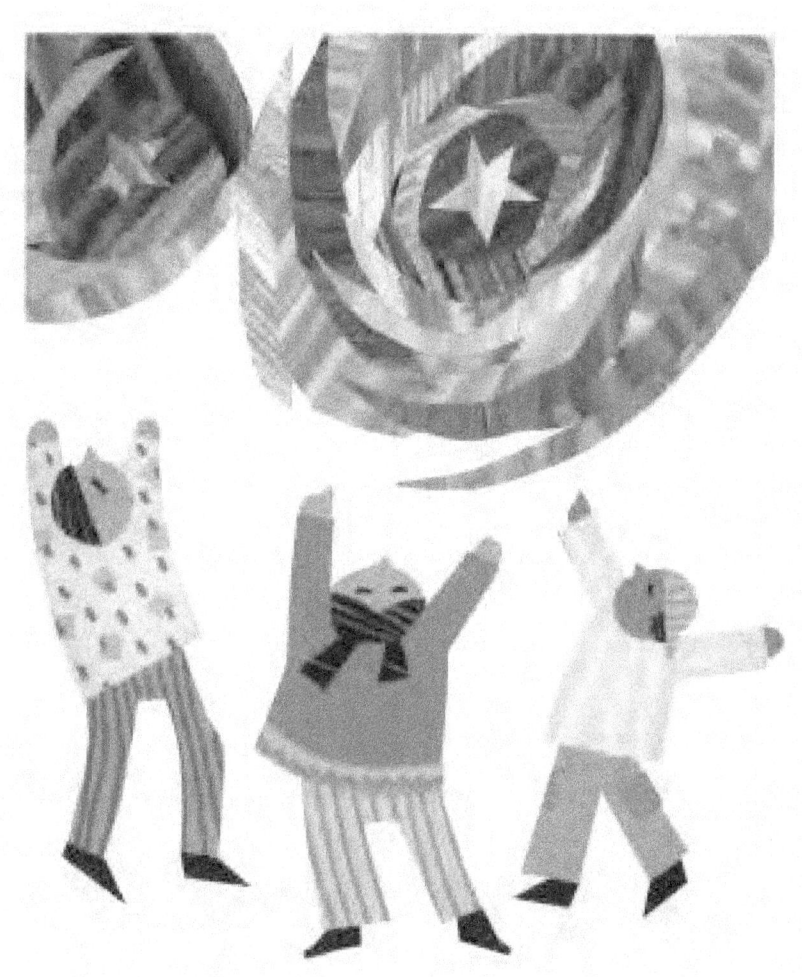

# CASE STUDY I: EPIDEMIOLOGY OF STDS: OUTBREAK INVESTIGATION

## Part I:

The investigation of an ongoing outbreak requires quick action and a systematic approach to help ensure that the investigation proceeds rapidly. The sequence of an outbreak investigation is outlined below.

### Steps of an Outbreak Investigation

1. Prepare for field work

2. Establish the existence of an outbreak

3. Verify the diagnosis

4. Define and identify cases

   a. Establish a case definition

   b. Identify and count cases

5. Perform descriptive epidemiology

6. Develop hypotheses

7. Evaluate hypotheses

8. Reconsider/refine hypotheses and execute further studies as necessary

   a. Additional epidemiologic studies

   b. Other types of studies (e.g., laboratory, environmental)

9. Implement control and prevention measures

10. Communicate findings

Source: CDC. Principles of epidemiology: an introduction to applied epidemiology and biostatistics. Atlanta (GA): Centers for Disease Control and Prevention; 1992.

Q1: The following table shows early syphilis (primary and secondary) rates for 1993–1997, for the city of Baltimore, Maryland, United States.

|  | 1993 | 1994 | 1995 | 1996 | 1997 |
|---|---|---|---|---|---|
| U.S. total | 10.3 | 7.9 | 6.3 | 4.3 | 3.2 |
| Maryland (state) | 7.2 | 6.5 | 11.0 | 14.4 | 17.6 |
| Baltimore (city) | 20.1 | 27.3 | 60.3 | 81.9 | 99.1 |

a) Divide into three small groups and let each group draw a line graph of the epidemic curve: one for the United States, one for Maryland, and one for Baltimore.

b) As a whole group, compare the epidemic curves. Would you say that, compared with the entire United States, there was a syphilis epidemic in Maryland? In Baltimore?

c) How much higher were syphilis rates in Baltimore than in the entire United States in 1993?

d) How much higher were syphilis rates in Baltimore than in the entire United States in 1997?

e) Assume that you are a health officer working in Baltimore. You have collected additional information on congenital syphilis and confirmed that since 1995 there has been a marked increase in congenital syphilis in Baltimore. You have information that confirms the epidemic. What additional steps will you take to investigate this outbreak?

## Part II:

Q2: Investigators have decided to ask two research questions:

- Has there been an increase in congenital syphilis in Baltimore during the 15-month study period?

- What factors are associated with the increase?

a) What type of study is needed to answer each of these questions—descriptive or analytic?

b) During the study period, 146 women were reported as having reactive syphilis serologies during pregnancy. The reporting forms for each of these women were reviewed by the study team. Of these 146 women, 56 were determined to have no active syphilis during pregnancy due to prior treatment, false positive serologies, or postpartum infection. What was the total number of women with active syphilis during pregnancy?

c) What two steps in the outbreak investigation have just been completed?

d) The investigators decided to conduct a case-control study to compare women with inadequately treated syphilis during pregnancy with those who were adequately treated for syphilis during pregnancy. Adequate therapy is defined as a stage-appropriate penicillin regimen started at least 30 days before delivery. The definition of inadequate therapy, then, includes no treatment, treatment started within 30 days of delivery, or treatment with no appropriate serologic response. Which of the pregnant women would be the most appropriate cases in this investigation and which would be the most appropriate controls?

e) The investigators found that 28 women had adequately treated syphilis and 62 had inadequately treated syphilis. What percentage of pregnant women with syphilis had adequately treated syphilis and what percentage had inadequately treated syphilis?

## Part III: Risk Factors

Q3: The following table summarizes some of the findings from the case control study:

|  | Cases | Controls |
| --- | --- | --- |
| **Mother's toxicology screen at delivery** |  |  |
| Cocaine positive | 22 (55%) | 11 (58%) |
| Opiate positive* | 17 (43%) | 2 (11%) |
| **Timing of syphilis diagnosis** |  |  |
| Third trimester* | 43 (74%) | 8 (29%) |
| **Had any syphilis education** | 6 (10%) | 5 (18%) |
| **Unwanted pregnancy*** | 23 (37%) | 4 (14%) |

* $P < .05$

a) Which risk factors were statistically significant?

b) After noting that late diagnosis was a significant risk factor for congenital syphilis, the investigators decided to examine the cases in further detail. They found that in 34 of the cases, women either had no prenatal care or initiated prenatal care after 28 weeks. What percentage of the cases were in this category?

c) The significant findings have implications for the importance of horizontal collaboration between STD and reproductive health providers. What are these implications?

The majority of these 34 women had contact with other providers (were in jail or had contact with social workers) who could have helped refer them into prenatal care at an earlier date.

## Part IV: Multivariate Analysis of Factors Associated With Congenital Syphilis

Q4: In further analyses, the investigators used only birth certificate data and compared two groups: 1) birth certificate data for the 38 black infants with congenital syphilis who were born in Baltimore in 1996 and 2) birth certificate data for the 5,966 black infants without congenital syphilis who were born in 1996 in Baltimore. They used logistic regression to adjust each risk factor for other risk factors in the statistical model. These results are shown below:

| Factor | Adjusted Odds Ratio (95% Confidence Interval) |
| --- | --- |
| **Prenatal care** | |
| Started first trimester | 0 (referent) |
| Started second trimester | 2.7 (0.9–8.0) |
| Started third trimester | 13.1 (4.2–40.7) |
| None | 12.0 (3.6–39.7)) |
| **Father's name missing** | 7.9 (3.1–19.8) |
| **Gravidity > 4** | 2.7 (1.1–6.8) |
| **Out-of-hospital delivery** | 12.7 (2.9–55.7) |

a) Which of the risk factors are statistically significant?

b) How would you interpret the findings regarding prenatal care?

# Part V: Implement Control Measures

At the start of this epidemic, Maryland state law required a first and third trimester syphilis test for pregnant women. Since there was no specification regarding timing of the third trimester test, many of these were performed at delivery—too late to prevent congenital syphilis.

Q5: Among pregnant women who entered prenatal care by 28 weeks, syphilis screening at 28 weeks could have prevented 18 cases of syphilis. What proportion of the total cases could be prevented by this intervention?

Q6: What recommendations should the agencies conducting this investigation make to legislators regarding timing of the third trimester syphilis test?

Note: The legislation for the state of Maryland was changed in January 1998 as a consequence of this investigation and now requires that the second syphilis test be conducted at 28 weeks of gestation or the first visit thereafter.

# ANSWERS

## Part I:

Q1:

a) (Line graphs of epidemic curves)

b) There appears to be an epidemic in Baltimore, but not in the entire state of Maryland.

c) Twice

d) About 33 times higher

e) Additional steps to investigate this outbreak:

- Verify diagnosis

- Count cases

- Describe the epidemic

- Test hypotheses

- Implement control measures

## Part II:

Q2:

a) A descriptive study is needed to answer the first question; an analytic study is needed to answer the second question.

b) 90

c) Diagnoses have been verified and cases have been counted.

d) The most appropriate cases would be pregnant women with inadequately treated syphilis and the most appropriate controls would be women with adequately treated syphilis.

e) Percentage of pregnant women with adequate treatment = 31% (28/90)
Percentage of pregnant women with inadequate treatment = 69% (62/90)

# Part III: Risk Factors

Q3:

    a) Significant findings:

- Cases were significantly more likely than controls to have a toxicology screening that was opiate-positive (43% versus 11%).

- Cases were significantly more likely than controls to have syphilis diagnosed during the third trimester (74% versus 29%).

- Cases were significantly more likely than controls to report that their pregnancy was unwanted (37% versus 14%).

    b) 55% (34/62)

    c) The need for close collaboration between STD clinicians and reproductive health clinicians is evident. Although the STD clinicians are the experts in the diagnosis and treatment of syphilis, reproductive health clinicians are the first group to see pregnant women for prenatal care, and the reproductive health clinicians are the group that could decrease unwanted pregnancy (thereby preventing congenital syphilis) by making modern family planning methods available.

# Part IV: Multivariate Analysis of Factors Associated With Congenital Syphilis

Q4:

    a) Significant findings from birth certificate data:

- Starting prenatal care in the third trimester, or having no prenatal care

- Father's name missing

- Gravidity of 4 or more

- Out-of-hospital delivery

    b) Two risk factors (no prenatal care and starting prenatal care in third trimester) have similar strength of association with congenital syphilis. It appears that starting prenatal care in the third trimester may be too late for adequately diagnosing and treating syphilis prior to delivery.

## Part V: Implement Control Measures

Q5: Proportion of the total cases preventable by intervention = 18/62 ≈ 29%.

Q6: The syphilis test should be conducted at 28 weeks of gestation, or at the first health care visit thereafter.

# CASE STUDY II

## EPIDEMIOLOGY OF STDs: QUESTIONNAIRE EXERCISE

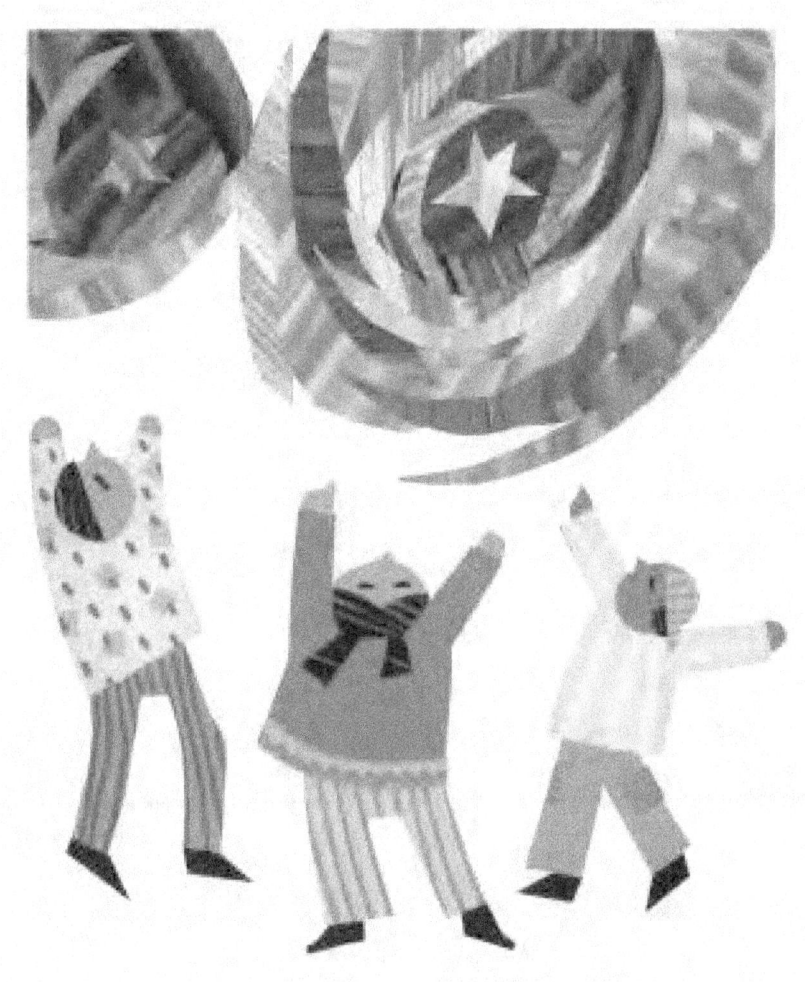

## CASE STUDY II: EPIDEMIOLOGY OF STDS: QUESTIONNAIRE EXERCISE

Your group is designing a study to evaluate the risk factors for syphilis in women under the age of 25 years who attend women's consultation clinics or dermatovenereology clinics. The following are the sexual behaviors you want to measure:

- Sexual activity

- Consistent condom use with regular partners

- Consistent condom use with casual partners

- Unprotected intercourse with regular partners

- Unprotected intercourse with casual partners

- Number of sex partners

- Exchanging sex for money

- Exchanging sex for drugs

- Use of intravenous drugs


1. Each group member should take several minutes to develop a question to measure one of the previous behaviors (5 minutes).

2. Each member of the workgroup should read his or her question to the group (5 minutes).

3. Group members can then work together to revise/improve each others' questions (10 minutes).

4. Attached are some sexual behavior questions that have been used previously in a variety of national surveys. (Although a discussion of questionnaire design is beyond the scope of this case study, it may help you to be aware that the SKIP pattern or other directions in CAPS and the numerical codes at the end of each response are used to facilitate and standardize interviewing and data entry.) Discuss how the questions should be modified to be culturally appropriate for use with patients in a dermatovenereology clinic or a women's consultation clinic.

1. During the past 12 months, have you had sex? By "sex" we mean only oral, vaginal, or anal sex.

   Yes ............................................................................. 1

   No ........................................................................ 2 SKIP to END

   Refused ..................................................................... 9

2. During the past 12 months, with how many different people have you had sex?

   Number ................................................................ ____

   Don't know/Not sure ...................................... 777

   Refused ............................................................ 999

3. During the past 12 months, have you had sex with only males, only females, or with both males and females. PLEASE MARK ONE BOX FOR THE BEST ANSWER

   Only males.................................................................. 1

   Only females ............................................................. 2

   Both males and females ............................................ 3

   Refused .................................................................... 9

4. I'm going to read you a list. When I'm done, please tell me if any of the situations apply to you. You don't need to tell me which one.

   • You have used intravenous drugs in the past year.

   • You have been treated for a sexually transmitted disease or venereal disease in the past year.

   • You tested positive for having HIV, the virus that causes AIDS.

   • You had anal sex without a condom in the past year.

   Do any of these situations apply to you?

   Yes ........................................................................... 1

   No ............................................................................ 2

   Don't know/Not sure ............................................. 7

   Refused ................................................................... 9

   [Note: The above question may be too nonspecific for use in high-risk populations. However, if direct comparison with a general population survey is desired, this question should probably be included and be followed or be replaced by the following more specific questions.]

5. During the past 12 months, have you used a needle to inject a drug that was not prescribed for you, or that you took only for the experience it caused?

Yes ................................................................. 1

No .................................................................. 2

Refused ........................................................... 9

6. During the past 12 months, has a doctor or nurse told you that you had a sexually transmitted disease, for example, herpes, gonorrhea, chlamydia, or genital warts?

Yes ................................................................. 1

No .................................................................. 2

Don't know/Not sure ...................................... 7

Refused ........................................................... 9

7. Have you ever been told that you were infected with the AIDS virus (HIV)?

Yes ................................................................. 1

No .................................................................. 2

Don't know/Not sure ...................................... 7

Refused ........................................................... 9

8. During the past 12 months, have you given drugs for sex or received drugs for sex? Remember to include only oral, vaginal, or anal sex.

Yes ................................................................. 1

No .................................................................. 2

Refused ........................................................... 9

9. During the past 12 months, have you given money for sex or received money for sex? Remember to include only oral, vaginal, or anal sex.

Yes ................................................................. 1

No .................................................................. 2

Refused ........................................................... 9

[Note: Some surveys have combined questions 8 and 9, for example: In the past 12 months, have you given or taken money or drugs in exchange for sex?]

SAY: Now, I would like you to think back to the last time you had sex. Remember that by "sex" we mean only oral, vaginal, or anal sex.

10. The last time you had sex, was a condom used?

Yes ............................................................1

No ............................................................2  SKIP TO
Question 13

Don't know/Not sure ...............................7

Refused ....................................................9

11. The last time you had sex with this partner, did either of you use a condom for:

11a. Oral sex

Yes ........................................................ 1

No ......................................................... 2

Don't know ........................................... 7

Did not have oral sex ........................... 8

Refused ................................................. 9

11b. Vaginal sex

Yes ........................................................ 1

No ......................................................... 2

Don't know ........................................... 7

Did not have vaginal sex ...................... 8

Refused ................................................. 9

11c. Anal sex

Yes ........................................................ 1

No ......................................................... 2

Don't know ........................................... 7

Did not have anal sex ........................... 8

Refused ................................................. 9

12. Was the condom used...

To prevent pregnancy ............................................. 1

To prevent diseases like syphilis, gonorrhea,
and AIDS ............................................................ 2

For both of these reasons ...................................... 3

For some other reason: Specify_____ 4

Don't know/Not sure ............................................ 7

Refused ................................................................ 9

SAY: Now I'm going to ask you some questions about the person
you last had sex with.

13. Is/was this person a man or a woman?

Man ...................................................................... 1

Woman .................................................................. 2

Refused ................................................................. 9

14. How long have you been having sex with this person?

Thirty days or less ................................................. 1

More than 30 days, but less than 6 months .......... 2

Six months or more ............................................... 3

Refused ................................................................. 9

15. Has this person ever injected (shot) drugs?

Yes ........................................................................ 1

No ......................................................................... 2

Don't know/Not sure ............................................. 7

Refused ................................................................. 9

16. Has this person ever had a sexually transmitted disease, for
example, herpes, gonorrhea, chlamydia, or genital warts?

Yes ........................................................................ 1

No ......................................................................... 2

Don't know/Not sure ............................................. 7

Refused ................................................................. 9

17. Does this person have the AIDS virus (HIV)?

    Yes ...................................................... 1

    No ....................................................... 2

    Don't know/Not sure ............................... 7

    Refused ................................................. 9

18. During the past 12 months, has this person given drugs for sex or received drugs for sex?

    Yes ...................................................... 1

    No ....................................................... 2

    Don't know/Not sure ............................... 7

    Refused ................................................. 9

19. During the past 12 months, has this person given money for sex or received money for sex?

    Yes ...................................................... 1

    No ....................................................... 2

    Don't know/Not sure ............................... 7

    Refused ................................................. 9

20. The last time you had sex with this person, had you been drinking alcohol before you had sex?

    Yes ...................................................... 1

    No ....................................................... 2

    Don't know/Not sure ............................... 7

    Refused ................................................. 9

21. The last time you had sex with this person, had you been using drugs like cocaine, heroin, crack, speed/crank, or marijuana before you had sex?

    Yes ...................................................... 1

    No ....................................................... 2

    Don't know/Not sure ............................... 7

    Refused ................................................. 9

    [Adapted from previous similar questions: "During the past 12 months, how often had you been using drugs like cocaine, heroin, crack, speed/crank, or marijuana before you had sex?" and "This most recent time you had sex, did either you or your partner use drugs to get high or intoxicated before or during sex?"]

22. The last time you had sex, was it with someone you are/were in an ongoing relationship with or who you consider(ed) to be your main sexual partner?

Yes ........................................................................1

No .....................................................................2 SKIP to END

Refused ................................................................9

[The following set of questions are the same as questions 10–22, but they are asked for the last time a person had sex with someone other than their main sexual partner. Since there is no known precedent for this method, its benefits and disadvantages should be considered prior to use.]

23. In the past 12 months, have you had sex with someone other than your main sexual partner?

Yes ........................................................................1

No .....................................................................2 SKIP to END

Refused .............................................................9 SKIP to END

SAY: The next couple of questions are about the last time you had sex with this other partner. Remember, by "sex" we mean oral, vaginal, or anal sex.

24. The last time you had sex with this person, was a condom used?

Yes ........................................................................1

No .....................................................................2 SKIP to Question 27

Don't know/Not sure ...........................................7

Refused ................................................................9

25. The last time you had sex with this person, was a condom used for:

25a. Oral sex

Yes ........................................................... 1

No ............................................................ 2

Don't know ............................................... 7

Did not have oral sex .................................. 8

Refused ..................................................... 9

25b. Vaginal sex

    Yes ................................................... 1

    No .................................................... 2

    Don't know ........................................ 7

    Did not have vaginal sex ........................ 8

    Refused ............................................. 9

25c. Anal sex

    Yes ................................................... 1

    No .................................................... 2

    Don't know ........................................ 7

    Did not have anal sex ........................... 8

    Refused ............................................. 9

26. Was the condom used...

    To prevent pregnancy ........................... 1

    To prevent diseases like syphilis, gonorrhea,
       and AIDS ..................................... 2

    For both of these reasons ...................... 3

    For some other reason: Specify_____ 4

    Don't know/Not sure ........................... 7

    Refused ............................................. 9

SAY: Now I'm going to ask you some questions about this person.

27. Is/was this person a man or a woman?

    Man .................................................. 1

    Woman .............................................. 2

    Refused ............................................. 9

28. How long have you been having sex with this person?

    Thirty days or less ............................... 1

    More than 30 days, but less than 6 months .......... 2

    Six months or more ............................. 3

    Refused ............................................. 9

29. Has this person ever injected drugs?

    Yes ........................................................................1

    No .........................................................................2

    Don't know/Not sure ..........................................7

    Refused ................................................................9

30. Has this person ever had a sexually transmitted disease, for example, herpes, gonorrhea, chlamydia, or genital warts?

    Yes ....................................................................... 1

    No ........................................................................ 2

    Don't know/Not sure ..........................................7

    Refused ................................................................9

31. Does this person have the AIDS virus (HIV)?

    Yes ........................................................................1

    No .........................................................................2

    Don't know/Not sure ..........................................7

    Refused ................................................................9

32. During the past 12 months, has this person given drugs for sex or received drugs for sex?

    Yes ...................................................................... 1

    No ....................................................................... 2

    Don't know/Not sure ..........................................7

    Refused ................................................................9

33. During the past 12 months, has this person given money for sex or received money for sex?

    Yes ........................................................................1

    No .........................................................................2

    Don't know/Not sure ..........................................7

    Refused ................................................................9

34. The last time you had sex with this person, had you been drinking alcohol before you had sex?

    Yes ....................................................... 1

    No .........................................................2

    Don't know/Not sure .......................................... 7

    Refused .................................................. 9

35. The last time you had sex with this person, had you been using drugs like cocaine, heroin, crack, speed/crank, or marijuana before you had sex?

    Yes ....................................................... 1

    No .........................................................2

    Don't know/Not sure .......................................... 7

    Refused .................................................. 9

As part of an initiative to address behavioral surveillance for HIV/STD prevention, the Behavioral Surveillance Workgroup at the National Center for HIV, STD, and TB Prevention, CDC has drafted a core set of sexual behavior questions. This module (including previous questions) is available for review at: http://www.cdc.gov/nchstp/od/core_workgroup/default.htm.

# APPENDIX A.

## OVERVIEW OF COMMON RTIS AND STDS

# APPENDIX A. OVERVIEW OF COMMON RTIs AND STDs

Adapted from: CDC. Family planning methods and practice: Africa. 2nd ed. Atlanta (GA): CDC; 1999.

| Disease (Pathogen) | Symptoms | Diagnosis | Treatment | Patient Instructions |
|---|---|---|---|---|
| **Bacterial vaginosis, Anaerobic vaginosis**<br><br>Clinical syndrome of anaerobic vaginal bacteria (e.g., Gardnerella vaginalis, Myco-plasma hominis, and other anaerobes) overgrowing normal lactobacilli | Excessive or foul-smelling vaginal discharge. Other signs include erythema, irritation, and intense itching of the external genitalia. Frequently assumed to be normal discharge by develop-ing world women. | *Presumptive diagnosis:* Typical symptoms of vulvovaginitis, elevated vaginal pH (> 4.7), and presence of clue cells in saline wet mount or gram stain of vaginal discharge. Diagnosis enhanced with fishy odor of vaginal discharge after addition of 1–2 drops of 10% potassium hydroxide (KOH). Cultures are not useful. Only symptomatic women need to be treated. Male sex partners do not. | *Recommended regimens:* Metronidazole 400–500 mg PO twice a day for 7 days *OR* Metronidazole 2 g PO once.<br><br>Metronidazole is contraindi-cated during the first trimester of pregnancy but may be used, if necessary, during the second and third trimesters. Data on alternative regimens are very limited. Clindamycin 300 mg PO twice a day for 7 days has been used successfully and this regimen would be safe in pregnancy. | Understand how to take or use any prescribed medications. Avoid drinking alcohol until 24 hours after completing metronidazole medication. |
| **Chancroid**<br><br>(Haemophilus ducreyi) | Frequently asymp-tomatic in women. Symptoms appear 3–10 days after infection. Typically a single (sometimes multiple) painful, irregularly-shaped genital ulcer. Ulcer is soft, and its base may be covered with grey purulent exudate. Ulcer usually on the penis or at entrance to vagina or anus. Ulcers usually disappear without treatment in about 1 month. Painful inguinal adenopathy (tender-ness of groin) in 50% of cases. | *Presumptive diagnosis:* Clinical presentation consistent with chan-croid, a unilateral bubo, or both. Diagnosis by exclusion of other STDs causing genital ulcers: negative darkfield microscopy or serologic testing (syphilis) *AND* inconsistent clinical presentation of ulcer(s) or negative culture (genital herpes).<br><br>*Definitive diagnosis:* Identification of *H. ducreyi* on special culture media. | *Recommended regimen:* Erythromycin 500 mg PO 3 times a day for 7 days.<br><br>*Alternative regimens:* Ciprofloxacin 500 mg PO once *OR* Ceftriaxone 250 mg IM once *OR* Spectinomycin 2 g IM once *OR* Trimethoprim (80 mg)/ Sulphamethoxazole (400 mg) 2 tablets twice a day for 7 days.<br><br>The latter regimen has been shown to be less effective in some parts of Africa and should only be used in areas where *in vitro* resistance rates are low and monitored regularly. Due to widespread resistance, tetracycline and penicillins should not be used. | Obtain HIV testing because genital ulcers are associated with HIV. Refer sex partners for treatment. Carefully clean ulcerative lesion(s) 3 times a day. Use condoms to prevent future infections. |

| Disease (Pathogen) | Symptoms | Diagnosis | Treatment | Patient Instructions |
|---|---|---|---|---|
| **Chlamydia**<br><br>(Chlamydia trachomatis) | Sexually transmitted infections caused by *C. trachomatis.* Symptoms usually appear 7–21 days after infection and include purulent cervical discharge or watery white or yellow urethral discharge. Other symptoms include spotting after sexual intercourse, pain on urination, and lower abdominal pain. Can lead to PID, ectopic pregnancy, and infertility in women and chlamydial ophthalmia and pneumonia in newborns. Often, men, and especially women, have asymptomatic infections. | *Presumptive diagnosis:* Diagnosis usually by exclusion, in the absence of culturing techniques. In symptomatic women, presence of yellow mucopurulent endocervical exudate. In asymptomatic women, presence of S10 PMN leukocytes per x 1,000 field on Gram's stain of endocervical mucus. In symptomatic men (with negative gonorrhea tests), white blood cells on Gram's stain of urethral discharge *OR* sexual exposure to an NGU-causing agent. In asymptomatic men (with negative gonorrhea tests), S4 PMN leukocytes per x 1,000 field on intraurethral smear.<br><br>*Definitive diagnosis:* Diagnosis by observed growth on cycloheximide-treated McCoy cells. Fluorescent monoclonal antibody stains or enzyme immunoassay tests may be available. Future use of DNA amplification techniques may increase sensitivity. | *Recommended regimens:* Doxycycline 100 mg PO twice a day for 7 days *OR* Tetracycline 500 mg PO 4 times a day for 7 days.<br><br>Tetracyclines are contraindicated during pregnancy.<br><br>*Alternative regimens (for patients in whom Tetracyclines are contraindicated or not tolerated):* Erythromycin 500 mg PO 4 times a day for 7 days *OR*, if Erythromycin is not tolerated, Sulfisoxazole 500 mg PO 4 times daily for 10 days. Equivalent doses of other sulphonamides may be used. Azythromycin 1 g PO once is effective treatment for chlamydia urethritis, but because its efficacy has not been proven in nongonococcal urethritis, it only should be used where a chlamydial etiology has been proven. This regimen is also expensive. (Gonorrhea resistance has been documented. This resistance, plus expense and side effects from a 2 g PO dose, make this regimen inadvisable for dual treatment.) | Sex partners must be treated. Use condoms to prevent future infections. |
| **Genital warts** (Condyloma acuminata)<br><br>**Human papillomavirus** (HPV) | Appear as single or multiple, soft, dry, painless, skin-colored growths around the vulvovaginal area, penis, anus, urethra, or perineum. In women, growths may occur on vaginal or cervical walls and not be noticed. Symptoms appear from one to several months after infection. HPV cannot be cured, even if warts disappear. Can cause cervical and other genital cancers in adults. | *Presumptive diagnosis:* By typical clinical presentation on the external genitalia or of koilocytosis on Pap smear specimens. Colposcopy may aid in diagnosis of certain cervical lesions. Exclude possibility of condyloma lata (flat, moist lesions) with darkfield microscopy or serologic tests for syphilis.<br><br>*Definitive diagnosis:* By biopsy, but usually un-necessary. Very atypical lesions, where neoplasia is a consider-ation, should be biopsied before therapy. Some warts in the anogenital area are associated with genital dysplasia or carcinoma. A Pap smear of cervical lesions shows typical cytologic changes. | *Regimens for external genital, perianal, vaginal warts:* (Physical) Cryotherapy with liquid nitrogen, solid carbon dioxide, or cryoprobe *OR* electro-surgery *OR* surgical removal.<br><br>(Chemical) Podophyllin, 10%–25% in compound tincture of benzoin should be applied to warts, avoiding normal tissue. Wash off warts thoroughly 1–4 hours after podophyllin appli-cation. Podophyllin should not be used for anal, urethral, oral, or cervical warts, and is contraindi-cated during pregnancy and lactation. *OR* Trichloroacetic acid (80%–90%) applied to warts weekly.<br><br>*Note:* Treatment of cervical warts should not start until a satisfactory cervical smear is obtained. Manage-ment should be carried out in consultation with an expert. | Sex partners do not need to be examined, as most are already infected. However, anogenital warts are contagious to uninfected sex partners. Use condoms to prevent infection to uninfected sex partners. Because HPV is incurable, warts can reappear after removal. |

| Disease (Pathogen) | Symptoms | Diagnosis | Treatment | Patient Instructions |
|---|---|---|---|---|
| **Gonorrhea** (Neisseria gonorrhoeae) | Symptoms usually appear 1–14 days after infection. Symptoms in men include pain on urination, increased frequency of urination, and yellow or white purulent urethral discharge. Up to 25% of infected men may be asymptomatic. Often asymptomatic in women. When present, symptoms include abnormal vaginal discharge, pain on urination, spotting after sexual intercourse, lower abdominal pain, and abnormal or painful menses. Infection can cause PID and sterility in women; urethritis, epididymitis, and sterility in men; and ophthalmia neonatorum in newborns. | *Presumptive diagnosis:* Microscopic identification of typical gram-negative intracellular diplococci on smear of urethral exudate (men) or endocervical material (women) *OR* growth on selective medium demonstrating typical colonial morphology, positive oxidase reaction, and typical Gram-stain morphology. *Definitive diagnosis:* Growth on selective medium demonstrating typical colonial morphology, positive oxidase reaction, and typical Gram-stain morphology, and confirmed by sugar utilization, coagglutination, or antigonococcal fluorescent antibody testing. | *Recommended regimens:* Ceftriaxone 125 or 250 mg IM once *OR* Cefixime 400 mg PO once *OR* Spectinomycin 2 g IM once *OR* Ofloxacin 400 mg PO once *OR* Ciprofloxacin 500 mg PO once (contraindicated in pregnancy); however, gonorrhea resistance to Ciprofloxacin has been documented. *Alternative regimens:* Kanamycin 2 g IM once *OR* Trimethoprim (80 mg)/ Sulphamethoxazole (400 mg), 10 tablets PO once daily for 3 days. Kanamycin and Trimethoprim/ sulphamethoxazole should only be used in regions where *N. gonorrhoeae* are susceptible and susceptibility is monitored at regular intervals. Second-line treatment with recommended drugs should be available. *PLUS* concurrent antichlamydial therapy such as Doxycycline 100 mg PO twice a day for 7 days. | Refer sex partners for examination and treatment. Avoid having sex until you and your partner(s) are completely cured. Understand how to take any prescribed oral medications. Use condoms to prevent future infections. |
| **Granuloma inguinale** (donovanosis) (Calymmato-bacterium granulomatis) | Symptoms appear 8–80 days after infection. Single or multiple nodules appear below the skin at the site of inoculation. Nodules break through to form granulomatous ulcers that are painless, bleed on contact, and enlarge slowly. In men, ulcers appear on glans and prepuce of penis. Women are frequently asymptomatic. | *Presumptive diagnosis:* Typical clinical presentation is sufficient. Resolution of lesions after antibiotic therapy supports diagnosis. *Definitive diagnosis:* Microscopic exam of scrapings of biopsy specimens from the ulcer margin reveals typical Donovan bodies. Tissue culture not feasible. | *Recommended regimen:* Trimethoprim (80 mg)/ Sulphamethoxazole (400 mg), 2 tablets twice a day for a minimum of 14 days and until lesions have completely re-epithelialized. *Alternative regimens:* Doxycycline 100 mg PO twice a day for 7 days *OR* Tetracycline 500 mg PO 4 times a day. | Understand how to take any prescribed oral medication. Refer sex partner(s) for examination. |

| Disease (Pathogen) | Symptoms | Diagnosis | Treatment | Patient Instructions |
|---|---|---|---|---|
| **Hepatitis B**<br><br>**Hepatitis B virus** (HBV) | Most HBV infections are clinically inapparent. When present, symptoms usually develop 1–9 months after contact and include serum sickness-like prodrome (skin eruptions, urticaria, arthralgias, arthritis), anorexia, vomiting, headache, fever, dark urine, jaundice, and moderate liver enlargement. Long-term complications include chronic hepatitis, cirrhosis, hepatocellular carcinoma, hepatic failure, and death. | *Presumptive diagnosis:* By typical clinical symptoms and exposure to a patient with presumed or definitive HBV infection.<br><br>*Definitive diagnosis:* Serodiagnosis of HBV infection. | No known cure. HBV is the only STD that has a vaccine. Vaccination of all newborn infants and adolescents is recommended. People with a recent STD and those with more than one sex partner in the previous 6 months also should receive HBV vaccine. | People at risk for sexual transmission of HBV are also at risk for HIV and other STDs. Condoms should be used to prevent future infections. Sex partners should be examined immediately. Vaccination can prevent infection among people exposed sexually to HBV if administered within 14 days of exposure. |
| **Herpes genitalis**<br><br>[Herpes simplex virus (types 1 & 2)] | HSV-2 is more common in genital disease. Single or multiple small vesicles, usually pruritic, on the genitalia. Vesicles spontaneously rupture to form shallow ulcers that may be very painful. Other symptoms include pain on intercourse, pain on urination, discharge, fever, and malaise. Initial symptoms appear 1–26 days after infection. First clinical occurrence is called first episode infection. Subsequent occurrences are usually milder and called recurrent episodes. HSV can be transmitted to newborns during vaginal delivery and cause neonatal herpes. Risk of transmission is highest with primary infection. | *Presumptive diagnosis:* Usually by clinical judgment. Likely when typical genital lesions are present or a pattern of recurrence has developed. Further supported by direct identification of multinucleated giant cells with intranuclear inclusions in a clinical specimen prepared by Papanicolaou or other serological techniques.<br><br>*Definitive diagnosis:* HSV tissue culture demonstrates the characteristic cytopathogenic effect following inoculation of a specimen from the cervix, urethra, or base of a genital lesion. | No known cure. Symptoms can be modified with Acyclovir treatment as soon as possible following onset of symptoms. Topical therapy with acyclovir produces only minimal shortening of the duration of symptomatic episodes and is not recommended.<br><br>*Recommended regimens:* First clinical episode: Acyclovir 200 mg PO 5 times a day for 5 days. (Treatment can be expected to reduce formation of new lesions, duration of pain, time to healing, and viral shedding; however, treatment will not influence the natural history of recurrent disease.)<br><br>*Recurrences:* Acyclovir 200 mg PO 5 times a day for 5 days. Suppression of recurrent outbreaks (> 6 per year): Acyclovir 200 mg 3 times a day PO continuously. | Keep involved area clean and dry. Refrain from sexual contact during symptomatic periods. Understand that HSV can also be transmitted during asymptomatic periods. Use condoms to minimize exposure to infection. |

| Disease (Pathogen) | Symptoms | Diagnosis | Treatment | Patient Instructions |
|---|---|---|---|---|
| **Lymphogranu-loma venereum** (LGV)<br><br>[Chlamydia trachomatis (types L1, L2, & L3)] | Genital lesion is a small, painless vesicle or nonindurated ulcer (often unnoticed). Inguinal adenopathy (buboes) follows 1–4 weeks after. Women may be asymptomatic, although some experience lower back pain and inguinal buboes. Symptoms appear after 3–12 days for genital lesion and after 10–30 days for inguinal bubo. LGV can cause cervicitis, urethritis, and enlargement of genitalia. | *Presumptive diagnosis:* Often diagnosed clinically and should be differentiated from chancroid. A titer of 1:64 on the LGV complement fixation test is considered diagnostic.<br><br>*Definitive diagnosis:* Isolation of *C. trachomatis* from appropriate specimen and confirmation of LGV immunotype, although such laboratory capabilities are not widely available. | *Recommended regimens:* Doxycycline 100 mg PO twice a day for 14 days *OR* Tetracycline 500 mg PO 4 times a day for 14 days.<br><br>*Alternative regimens:* Erythromycin 500 mg PO 4 times a day for 14 days *OR* Sulphadiazine 1 g PO 4 times a day for 14 days. Other sulphonamides can be used in equivalent doses.<br><br>Fluctuant lymph nodes should be aspirated as needed. Incision and drainage or excision of nodes will delay healing and are contraindicated. | Understand how to take any prescribed oral medications. Refer sex partner(s) for examination as soon as possible. |

| Disease (Pathogen) | Symptoms | Diagnosis | Treatment | Patient Instructions |
|---|---|---|---|---|
| **Pelvic Inflammatory Disease** (PID)<br><br>Polymicrobial etiology: combinations of *N. gonorrhoeae*, *C. trachomatis*, anaerobic bacteria, facultative gram-negative rods, *M. hominis*, and other microbial agents. | Spectrum of inflammatory disorders of upper genital tract of women. Many women have atypical or no symptoms. Symptoms include pain and tenderness of the lower abdomen, cervix, uterus, and adnexae. Other possible symptoms are elevated white blood cell count, dyspareunia, vaginal discharge, menometrorrhagia, dysuria, pain with menses, fever, chills, and sometimes nausea and vomiting. Risk of PID increased by multiple sex partners, history of PID, or recent insertion of intrauterine device. PID can cause infertility, chronic pain, pelvic abscess, and ectopic pregnancy. | *Presumptive diagnosis:* By typical clinical symptoms if other serious conditions, such as acute appendicitis or ectopic pregnancy, can be excluded. Diagnosis often based on imprecise clinical findings.<br><br>*Definitive diagnosis:* Through direct visualization of inflamed (edema, hyperemia, or tubal exudate) fallopian tube(s) during laparoscopy or laparotomy. Cultures of tubal exudate may be helpful. | Because the causative organisms are usually unknown at the start of therapy, use regimens effective against a broad range of pathogens.<br><br>*Inpatient therapy:*<br>Recommended regimens:<br>1. Ceftriaxone 500 mg IM once daily *PLUS* Doxycycline 100 mg PO or IV twice a day *OR* Tetracycline 500 mg PO 4 times a day *PLUS* Metronidazole 400–500 mg PO *OR* IV twice a day or Chloramphenicol 500 mg PO or IV 4 times a day.<br>2. Clindamycin 900 mg IV 8 hourly *PLUS* Gentamicin 1.5 mg/kg IV 8 hourly.<br>3. Ciprofloxacin 500 mg PO twice a day *OR* Spectinomycin 1 g IM 4 times a day *PLUS* Doxycycline 100 mg PO or IV 2 times a day *OR* Tetracycline 500 mg 4 times a day *PLUS* Metronidazole 400–500 mg PO or IV twice a day *OR* Chloramphenicol 500 mg PO or IV 4 times a day.<br><br>Duration of therapy should be at least 2 days after the patient has improved. This treatment should be followed by either Doxycycline 100 mg PO twice a day *OR* tetracycline 500 mg PO 4 times a day, both for 14 days.<br><br>*Ambulatory therapy:*<br>Recommended regimens:<br>Single-dose therapy for uncomplicated gonorrhea (e.g., Ceftriaxone) *PLUS* Doxycycline 100 mg PO twice a day for 14 days *OR* Ofloxacin, 400 mg PO twice a day for 14 days *PLUS* Metronidazole 500 mg PO twice a day for 14 days.<br><br>Alternative regimens (in absence of single-dose gonorrhea therapy) Trimethoprim (80 mg)/ Sulphamethoxazole (400 mg) 10 tablets PO once a day for 3 days and then 2 tablets twice a day for 10 days *PLUS* Doxycycline 100 mg PO twice daily or Tetracycline 500 mg PO 4 times a day for 14 days *PLUS* Metronidazole 400–500 mg PO twice a day for 14 days. | Refer sex partner(s) for evaluation and treatment. Many sex partners are infected but asymptomatic. Avoid sexual activity until you and your partner(s) are cured. Understand how to take any prescribed oral medications. Use condoms to prevent future infections. |

| Disease (Pathogen) | Symptoms | Diagnosis | Treatment | Patient Instructions |
|---|---|---|---|---|
| **Syphilis** (Treponema pallidum) | *Primary stage:* Classical symptom is a chancre (indurated painless ulcer) at the site of exposure (e.g., vulva, cervix, penis, mouth, or anus). Internal lesions in women may not be detected. Lesion heals within a few weeks without treatment. Symptoms appear 10–90 days after infection. Differential diagnosis for all genital lesions should include syphilis.<br><br>*Secondary stage:* If primary stage untreated, symptoms will appear in a few weeks, including a highly variable skin rash (especially on palms of hands and soles of feet), general lymph node enlargement, condyloma lata, hair loss, and fever and malaise. Symptoms last several weeks to months and will disappear even without treatment.<br><br>*Latent:* No clinical signs of infection. Early syphilis (infectious) defined as primary, secondary, or latent syphilis of less than 2 years' duration. Late syphilis defined as latent syphilis of more than 2 years' duration or syphilis of unknown duration. Syphilis infection can cause congenital syphilis and late syphilis (including neuro-syphilis, cardiovascular syphilis, and localized gumma formation). | *Presumptive diagnosis:* *Primary stage:* By identification of typical lesion(s) and either 1) a positive darkfield exam; 2) fluorescent antibody techniques in material from a chancre, regional lymph node, or other lesion; 3) the presence of a serologic test for syphilis (STS) titer at least four-fold greater than the last; or 4) patient's exposure to syphilis within 90 days of lesion onset.<br><br>*Secondary stage:* Diagnosis through typical clinical presentation of symptoms and a strongly reactive STS. Condyloma lata will be darkfield positive.<br><br>*Latent stage:* Periods of infection with strongly reactive STS, but no clinical signs of infection.<br><br>*Definitive diagnosis:* Through identification of *T. pallidum* with darkfield microscopy or fluorescent antibody technique for primary and secondary syphilis. No definitive diagnosis for latent syphilis. | *Early syphilis (primary, second-ary, or latent syphilis of not more than 2 years' duration):*<br><br>*Recommended regimen:* Benzathine penicillin G 2.4 million units IM once (often given as two injections at separate sites).<br><br>*Alternative regimen:* Aqueous procaine penicillin G 1.2 million units IM daily for 10 consecutive days.<br><br>*Late latent and late benign syphilis (latent syphilis of indeterminate length or of more than 2 years' duration):*<br><br>*Recommended regimen:* Benzathine penicillin G 7.2 million units total, adminis-tered as 2.4 million units IM given 1 week apart for 3 consecutive weeks.<br><br>*Alternative regimen:* Aqueous procaine penicillin G 1.2 million units IM daily for 20 consecutive days.<br><br>*Neurosyphilis:* Recommended regimen: Aqueous crystalline penicillin G 12–24 million units total, administered as 2–4 million units every 4 hours IV for 14 days.<br><br>*Alternative regimen:* Aqueous procaine penicillin G 1.2 million units IM daily, *AND* probenecid 500 mg PO 4 times a day, both for 10–14 days.<br><br>*Penicillin-allergic patients:* Doxycycline 100 mg PO 2 times a day for 14 days (if early syphilis) or for 28 days (if late syphilis).<br><br>*Penicillin-allergic pregnant women:* Erythromycin 500 mg PO 4 times a day for 14 days. | Obtain testing for HIV infection because genital ulcers may facilitate HIV infection. Return for follow-up serologies. Understand how to take any prescribed oral medications. Avoid sexual activity until you and your partner(s) are cured. Use condoms to prevent future infections. |

| Disease (Pathogen) | Symptoms | Diagnosis | Treatment | Patient Instructions |
|---|---|---|---|---|
| Trichomoniasis<br><br>(Trichomonas vaginalis) | Excessive, frothy, green or yellow vaginal discharge, with foul odor. Itching, erythema, edema, pain on urination, and pain on intercourse also may occur. Some women may have no symptoms. Men are usually without symptoms, but may have urethritis, balanitis, cutaneous lesions on penis, pain on urination, and itching. Recurrent infections are common. | Diagnosis when a vaginal culture or fluorescent antibody is positive for *T. vaginalis* OR typical motile trichomonads are identified in a saline wet mount of vaginal discharge. Trichomonads found by Pap smear are not diagnostic of active infection. | *Recommended regimens:* Metronidazole 2 g PO once.<br><br>*Alternative regimen:* Metronidazole 400–500 mg PO twice a day for 7 days.<br><br>Metronidazole is contraindicated in the first trimester of pregnancy but may be used during the second and third trimesters. There is no evidence that other 5-nitro-imidazoles are superior to metronidazole, but they may be used when dictated by availability. Asymptomatic women should be treated with the same regimen as symptomatic women. *OR* Sulphadiazine 1 g PO 4 times a day for 14 days. Other sulphonamides can be used in equivalent doses.<br><br>Fluctuant lymph nodes should be aspirated as needed. Incision and drainage or excision of nodes will delay healing and are contraindicated. | Understand how to take or use any prescribed medications. Use condoms to prevent future infections. Avoid drinking alcohol until 24 hours after completing metronidazole therapy. Both asymptomatic and symptomatic male partners should be treated. |
| Vulvovaginal candidiasis<br><br>(Candida albicans) | Candida are normal flora of skin and vagina and not considered sexually transmitted infections. Clinical presentation varies from no signs or symptoms to itching, irritation, or pain of the external genitalia. Type of symptoms does not distinguish microbial etiology. Men may develop urethritis, balanitis, or cutaneous penile lesions. Recurrent infections are common. Persistent candidiasis may indicate HIV. | *Presumptive diagnosis:* By typical clinical symptoms of vulvo-vaginitis and microscopic identification of yeast forms or hyphae in Gram stain or KOH wet-mount preparations of vaginal discharge.<br><br>*Definitive diagnosis:* By positive culture for *C. albicans* (or other Candida species) in symptomatic women. Cultures may detect clinically insignificant infections (should not be treated) and are not recommended. | *Recommended regimens:* Miconazole or Clotrimazole, 200 mg intravaginally daily for 3 days *OR* Clotrimazole 500 mg intravaginally once, *OR* Nystatin 100,000 units intravaginally daily for 14 days. | Understand how to take or use any prescribed medications. Wear a sanitary pad to protect clothing and change pads frequently. Continue taking medicine even during menses. |

# APPENDIX B.

# EVALUATING DIAGNOSTIC TESTS

# Appendix B. Evaluating Diagnostic Tests

Adapted from: Greenberg RS, Daniels SR, Flanders WD, Eley JW, Boring JR. Medical epidemiology. 2nd ed. Stamford (CT): Appleton and Lange; 1996. p. 75–85.
Hennekens CH, Buring JE. Screening. In: Mayrent SL, editor. Epidemiology in medicine. Boston: Little, Brown and Company; 1987. p. 327–47.

The purpose of **diagnostic testing** is to determine the presence or absence of a particular condition. The process of testing to detect disease at its earliest stages among asymptomatic people in the general population is called **screening**. At other times, diagnostic tests are used in order to confirm a diagnosis among people with existing signs or symptoms of illness. In general, diagnostic and screening tests are evaluated by calculating their **sensitivity** or **specificity**. Sensitivity indicates how good a test is at identifying the disease, and specificity indicates how good a test is at identifying those who are free of disease.

Consider a test that has only positive or negative results. When evaluating a diagnostic test, four situations are possible: a) a **true positive** result, where the test is positive and the patient has the disease; b) a **false positive** result, where the test is positive but the patient does not have the disease; c) a **false negative** result, where the test is negative but the patient has the disease; and d) a **true negative** result, where the test is negative and the patient does not have the disease (see diagram below). The best diagnostic tests are those with few false positives and false negatives *(32)*.

**"Truth" or Gold Standard**

| Test Result | | disease | no disease |
|---|---|---|---|
| | positive | **a**<br>true positive | **b**<br>false positive |
| | negative | **c**<br>false negative | **d**<br>true negative |

Sensitivity and specificity are measures used to describe the accuracy of a test.

# Sensitivity

*Definition.* Sensitivity is defined as the percentage of people with the disease of interest who have positive test results.

$$\text{Sensitivity} = \frac{\text{True positives}}{\text{True positives} + \text{False negatives}} \times 100$$

$$= \frac{a}{a + c} \times 100$$

*Use and Interpretation.* The greater the sensitivity of a test, the more likely that the test will detect persons with the disease of interest. Tests with high sensitivity are useful clinically to rule out a disease; when sensitivity is high, there can be confidence in a negative test result.

# Specificity

*Definition.* Specificity is defined as the percentage of people without the disease of interest who have negative test results.

$$\text{Specificity} = \frac{\text{True negatives}}{\text{False positives} + \text{True negatives}} \times 100$$

$$= \frac{d}{b + d} \times 100$$

*Use and Interpretation.* The greater the specificity, the more likely that people without the disease of interest will not be identified by the test. Thus, highly specific tests are often used to confirm the presence of a disease.

The value of a diagnostic test depends not only on its sensitivity and specificity, but also on the prevalence of the disease in the population being tested. As the prevalence of a disease decreases, it becomes less likely that someone with a positive test actually has the disease and more likely that the test represents a false positive. Therefore, the rarer a disease, the more specific a test must be in order to be clinically useful. On the other hand, the more common a disease, the more sensitive the test must be to be clinically useful. Otherwise, a negative test is likely to represent a false negative.

# Prevalence

*Definition.* The prevalence of a disease is defined as the number of existing cases of the disease per total population at a given point in time.

$$\text{Prevalence} = \frac{\text{Number of existing cases of the disease of interest}}{\text{Total population}} \times 100$$

$$= \frac{a + c}{a + b + c + d} \times 100$$

*Use and Interpretation.* Prevalence can be thought of as the status of the disease in a population at a point in time and is sometimes referred to as point prevalence. The denominator includes the total population (for example, all women of reproductive age, both with and without the disease of interest).

The **predictive value positive and negative** are measures that directly address the estimation of probability of disease. Because it incorporates information on both the test and the population being tested, predictive value is a good measure of overall clinical usefulness.

# Predictive value positive

*Definition.* The predictive value positive (PV+) is the probability that a person with a positive test result actually has the disease.

$$PV+ = \frac{\text{True positives}}{\text{True positives} + \text{False positives}} \times 100$$

$$= \frac{a}{a + b} \times 100$$

*Use and Interpretation.* The PV+ is the proportion of people with positive test results who actually have the disease. This measure allows one to estimate how likely it is that the disease of interest is present if the test is positive.

## Predictive value negative

*Definition.* The predictive value negative (PV–) is the probability that a person with a negative test result does not have the disease.

$$PV- \quad = \frac{\text{True negatives}}{\text{False negatives} + \text{True negatives}} \times 100$$

$$= \frac{d}{c + d} \times 100$$

*Use and Interpretation.* The PV– is the proportion of people with negative test results who are free of disease; in other words, it is the probability of the disease being absent if the test is negative.

# REFERENCES

1. Wasserheit JN, Holmes KK. Reproductive tract infections: challenges for international health policy, programs, and research. In: Germain A, Holmes KK, Piot P, Wasserheit JN, editors. Reproductive tract infections: global impact and priorities for women's reproductive health. New York: Plenum Press; 1992. p. 7–33.

2. Rowley J, Berkley S. Sexually transmitted diseases. In: Murray CJL, Lopez AD, editors. Health dimensions of sex and reproduction. Boston: Harvard University Press; 1998. p. 19–110.

3. Adler MW. Sexually transmitted diseases control in developing countries. Genitourin 1996;72(2):83–8.

4. Brunham RC, Holmes KK, Embree JE. Sexually transmitted diseases in pregnancy. In: Holmes KK, Mardh P, Sparling PF, Wiesner PJ, Cates W, Lemon SM, et al., editors. Sexually transmitted diseases. New York: McGraw-Hill; 1990. p. 771–801.

5. CDC. Family planning methods and practice: Africa. 2nd ed. Atlanta (GA): United States Department of Health and Human Services, CDC; 1999.

6. Aral SO. Sexual behavior as a risk factor for sexually transmitted disease. In: Germain A, Holmes KK, Piot P, Wasserheit JN, editors. Reproductive tract infections: global impact and priorities for women's reproductive health. New York: Plenum Press; 1992. p. 185–98.

7. Cates W Jr. Reproductive tract infections. In: Hatcher RA, Trussell J, Stewart F, et al., editors. Contraceptive technology. New York: Ardent Media, Inc.; 1998. p. 179–210.

8. Schulz KF, Schulte JM, Berman SM. Maternal health and child survival: opportunities to protect both women and children from the adverse consequences of reproductive tract infections. In: Germain A, Holmes KK, Piot P, Wasserheit JN, editors. Reproductive tract infections: global impact and priorities for women's reproductive health. New York: Plenum Press; 1992. p. 145–82.

9. USAID. Integration of family planning/MCH with HIV/STD prevention. Washington: USAID; December 1998.

10. World Health Organization. Integrating STI management into family planning services: what are the benefits? Geneva, Switzerland: World Health Organization; 1999.

11. Wilkinson D, Ndovela N, Harrison A, Lurie M, Connolly C, Sturm AW. Family planning services in developing countries: an opportunity to treat asymptomatic and unrecognised genital tract infections? Genitourin 1997;73(6):558–60.

12. Finelli L, St. Louis ME, Gunn RA, Crissman CE. Epidemiologic support to state and local sexually transmitted disease control programs. Perceived need and availability. The Field Epidemiology Network for STDs (FENS). Sex Transm Dis 1998;25(3):132–6.

13. Catchpole MA. The role of epidemiology and surveillance systems in the control of sexually transmitted diseases. Genitourin 1996;72(5):321–9.

14. Gerbase AC, Rowley JT, Heymann DHL, Berkley SFB, Piot P. Global prevalence and incidence estimates of selected curable STDs. Sex Transm Infec 1998;74(Suppl 1):S12–S16.

15. Hook EW. Approaches to sexually transmitted disease control in North America and Western Europe. In: Wasserheit JN, Aral SO, Holmes KK, editors. Research issues in human behavior and sexually transmitted diseases in the AIDS era. Washington: American Society of Microbiology; 1991. p. 269–80.

16. Anderson RM. The transmission dynamics of sexually transmitted diseases: the behavioral component. In: Wasserheit JN, Aral SO, Holmes KK, editors. Research issues in human behavior and sexually transmitted diseases in the AIDS era. Washington: American Society of Microbiology; 1991. p. 38–60.

17. Padian NS, Shiboski SC, Hitchcock PJ. Risk factors for acquisition of sexually transmitted diseases and development of complications. In: Wasserheit JN, Aral SO, Holmes KK, editors. Research issues in human behavior and sexually transmitted diseases in the AIDS era. Washington: American Society of Microbiology; 1991. p. 83–96.

18. World Health Organization. Monitoring reproductive health: selecting a short list of national and global indicators. World Health Organization; 1997.

19. The Evaluation Project. Indicators for reproductive health program evaluation: final report of the subcommittee on STD/HIV. Chapel Hill (NC): Carolina Population Center, University of North Carolina; 1995.

20. Borisenko K. STD surveillance in the Russian Federation. STD AIDS 1998;9(Suppl 1):15.

21. Mayaud P, Msuya W, Todd J, Kaatano G, West B, Begkoyian G, et al. STD rapid assessment in Rwandan refugee camps in Tanzania. Genitourin 1997;73(1):33–8.

22. Webster LA. Analyzing STD surveillance data. Step 3: measures of disease frequency. CDC Division of STD/HIV Prevention Information Systems newsletter. Atlanta (GA): Centers for Disease Control and Prevention; 1993.

23. Dallabetta GA, Gerbase AC, Holmes KK. Problems, solutions, and challenges in syndromic management of sexually transmitted diseases. Sex Transm Infec 1998;74(Suppl 1):S1–S11.

24. Cates W Jr. A risk assessment tool for integrated reproductive health services. Fam Plann Perspect 1997;29(1):41–3.

25. Morrison CS, Sekadde-Kigondu C, Miller WC, Weiner DH, Sinei SK. Use of sexually transmitted disease risk assessment algorithms for selection of intrauterine device candidates. Contraception 1999;59(2):97–106.

26. Pettifor A, Walsh J, Wilkins V, Raghunathan P. How effective is syndromic management of STDs?: a review of current studies. Sex Transm Dis 2000;27:371–85.

27. Aral SO, Holmes KK. Epidemiology of sexual behavior and sexually transmitted diseases. In: Holmes KK, Mardh P, Sparling PF, Wiesner PJ, Cates W, Lemon SM, et al., editors. Sexually transmitted diseases. New York: McGraw-Hill; 1990. p. 19–36.

28. Friis RH, Sellars TA. Practical applications of epidemiology. In: Friis RH, Sellars TA. Epidemiology for public health practice. Gaithersburg (MD): Aspen Publishers; 1996. p. 60–1.

29. CDC. Sexually transmitted diseases treatment guidelines 2002. MMWR 2002;51(No. RR-6).

30. Dunlop JB, Segal S. Preface. In: Germain A, Holmes KK, Piot P, Wasserheit JN, editors. Reproductive tract infections: global impact and priorities for women's reproductive health. New York: Plenum Press; 1992.

31. World Health Organization. Progress in human reproduction research: reducing the impact of reproductive tract infections. No. 47. Geneva, Switzerland: World Health Organization; 1998.

32. Browner WS, Newman TB, Cummings SR. Designing a new study: III. Diagnostic tests. In: Hulley SB, Cummings SR, editors. Designing clinical research. Baltimore (MD): Williams and Wilkins; 1998. p. 89–91.